OBSTETRICS AND GYNECOLOGY ADVANCES

UTERINE FIBROIDS

FROM DIAGNOSIS TO TREATMENT

OBSTETRICS AND GYNECOLOGY ADVANCES

Additional books and e-books in this series can be found on Nova's website under the Series tab.

OBSTETRICS AND GYNECOLOGY ADVANCES

UTERINE FIBROIDS

FROM DIAGNOSIS TO TREATMENT

**MARCO MITIDIERI
SAVERIO DANESE
AND
ELISA PICARDO
EDITORS**

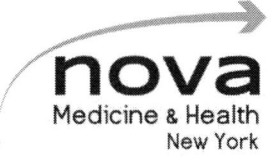

Copyright © 2021 by Nova Science Publishers, Inc.

All rights reserved. No part of this book may be reproduced, stored in a retrieval system or transmitted in any form or by any means: electronic, electrostatic, magnetic, tape, mechanical photocopying, recording or otherwise without the written permission of the Publisher.

We have partnered with Copyright Clearance Center to make it easy for you to obtain permissions to reuse content from this publication. Simply navigate to this publication's page on Nova's website and locate the "Get Permission" button below the title description. This button is linked directly to the title's permission page on copyright.com. Alternatively, you can visit copyright.com and search by title, ISBN, or ISSN.

For further questions about using the service on copyright.com, please contact:
Copyright Clearance Center
Phone: +1-(978) 750-8400   Fax: +1-(978) 750-4470   E-mail: info@copyright.com

NOTICE TO THE READER

The Publisher has taken reasonable care in the preparation of this book, but makes no expressed or implied warranty of any kind and assumes no responsibility for any errors or omissions. No liability is assumed for incidental or consequential damages in connection with or arising out of information contained in this book. The Publisher shall not be liable for any special, consequential, or exemplary damages resulting, in whole or in part, from the readers' use of, or reliance upon, this material. Any parts of this book based on government reports are so indicated and copyright is claimed for those parts to the extent applicable to compilations of such works.

Independent verification should be sought for any data, advice or recommendations contained in this book. In addition, no responsibility is assumed by the Publisher for any injury and/or damage to persons or property arising from any methods, products, instructions, ideas or otherwise contained in this publication.

This publication is designed to provide accurate and authoritative information with regard to the subject matter covered herein. It is sold with the clear understanding that the Publisher is not engaged in rendering legal or any other professional services. If legal or any other expert assistance is required, the services of a competent person should be sought. FROM A DECLARATION OF PARTICIPANTS JOINTLY ADOPTED BY A COMMITTEE OF THE AMERICAN BAR ASSOCIATION AND A COMMITTEE OF PUBLISHERS.

Additional color graphics may be available in the e-book version of this book.

Library of Congress Cataloging-in-Publication Data

ISBN: 978-1-53619-184-4

Published by Nova Science Publishers, Inc. † New York

CONTENTS

Preface		vii
Chapter 1	Imaging Features of Myometrium and Uterine Masses *Silvia Gemmiti, Houssein El Hajj,* *Chiara Benedetto,* *Stephanie Anne Sophie Gentile* *and Donatella Tota*	1
Chapter 2	Impact, Management, and Treatment of Uterine Myomas in Infertile Couples *Andrea Carosso, Alessandro Ruffa,* *Noemi Mercaldo, Bernadette Evangelisti* *and Alberto Revelli*	17
Chapter 3	Uterine Fibroids and Pregnancy: Last Insights *Alessandra Carosi, Giovanni Ruspa* *and Marta Tosi*	47
Chapter 4	Medical Treatment of Uterine Fibroids *Maria Grazia Baù and Alessandra Surace*	61

Chapter 5	Surgical Treatment for Uterine Fibroids *Livio Leo, Stephanie Challancin,* *Raphael Thomasset and Nicole Brunod*	71
Chapter 6	Postoperative Care After Myomectomy Surgery *Chiara Ferrari and Giuseppina Poppa*	109
Chapter 7	Uterine Artery Embolization: The Interventional Radiologist Point of View *Andrea Paladini, Pietro Danna,* *Massimiliano Cernigliaro,* *Giuseppe Guzzardi and Alessandro Carriero*	119
Chapter 8	Uterine Smooth Muscle Tumor of Uncertain Malignant Potential *Margerita Goia, Maria Giulia Disanto,* *Domenico Ferraioli and Andrea Palicelli*	135
About the Editors		147
Index		151

PREFACE

Uterine fibroids (UFs) are benign masses that develop from the smooth muscle cells and connective tissue of the wall of the uterus under the influence of genetic and / or hormonal stimuli.

These benign tumors are postulated to arise from a single, genetically altered, mesenchymal cell under the influence of gonadal hormones namely progesterone and 17β-estradiol. Particularly, African-American women are reported to have a higher leiomyoma incidence (80% versus 70%), with moresevere clinical symptoms, compared to Caucasians. Understanding their pathogenesis and molecular classification may facilitate development of effective targeted treatment options of this very common disease. Therefore, finding effective and improved therapeutical options is considered to be crucial for overcoming this major public health problem. But to find a novel therapy is usually strictly linked to an important step that is to explore the molecular basis of fibroids to understand and target the underlying specific pathophysiological pathways. Genetic factors have been implicated to play an important role in the development of fibroids through twin and familial aggregation studies, as well as through the observations of ethnic disparities in the incidence and clinical presentation of fibroids as exemplified by black women having increased prevalence, more severe symptoms, and earlier age of onset in comparison to white women. Research has to clarify the role of constitutional genetic variants, somatic alterations, and epigenetic mechanisms as challenging categories to identify novel pharmacological therapeutic approach for miomas. Epidemiologic data report that leiomyomata are virtually non existent prior to menarche and typically have an indolent course following menopause, strongly implicating gonadal hormones in the induction and maintenance of this disease process. Estimates say that 20 to 80% of women experience them throughout life, and are the most common form of benign cancer in childbearing age.

The annual societal cost for fibroids is estimated up to 34 billion dollars, calculated through combined expenditures for medical management of symptomatic fibroids, lost work attributable to diagnosis of fibroids, and obstetrical complications of fibroids In Italy, for example, they afflict 3 million women. Not all fibroids are symptomatic, so much so that they are often identified only during gynecological check-ups. In a certain percentage of patients, however, they can compromise the quality of life, causing abnormal intermenstrual bleeding and abundant flow, acute and chronic pelvic pain and, especially if voluminous, urination and defecation disorders (the mass presses on the bladder and on the intestine). Surgery has no more been the only therapeutic solution for some decades, since hormonal therapies have been introduced and proposed for myoma therapy. The use of medical treatment for myomas has largely grown in the last years, in particular women could be stratified into four categories according their wishes about treatment: women who would refuse surgery because of different reasons (such as fertility sparing or approaching menopause), women who wish postpone or women that are not candidates for surgery, or women already undergone to surgery with a preventive purpose. Myomectomy provides temporary reduction in uterine volume but is associated with a risk of recurrence estimated to be 11% with removal of a solitary fibroid and 26%or greater when multiple fibroids are removed over a10–30-month time period. Several therapeutic options are available for treating these patients that are confirmed to be safe and effective in reducing the symptoms and the size of the fibroids, avoiding or postponing surgery and preserving fertility. And the benefits are not limited to patients: as cost-effectiveness studies confirm, medical treatment proves to be the most advantageous therapeutic option also from a pharmacoeconomic point of view, with savings for the national health system estimated at around 45 million euro per year

Various surgical and medical options are currently available to manage symptomatic uterine fibroids. The choice of the appropriate therapeutic approach for UFs depends on several factors, including women's age, parity, childbearing aspirations and wish to preserve fertility, extent and severity of symptoms, size, number and location of myomas, risk of malignancy and proximity to menopause. Surgical treatment (hysterectomy and myomectomy) has long been the standard for symptomatic fibroids. Pharmacological therapy can also be used as an alternative to surgery or as a pre-operative ancillary to improve and optimize surgical outcomes by reducing size of myomas and/or uterine bleeding. It may be used as 'stand-alone' treatment for temporary short-term relief of symptoms, such as in the case of women with symptomatic fibroids in the pre-menopausal years or in patients not suitable for surgery due to medical reasons.

Because gonadal hormones induce, and maintain, leiomyoma growth via the production of an aberrant extracellular matrix (ECM), much research has focused on the development of medical agents to circumvent steroidal influence in an effort to reduce the burden of disease.These medications include centrally acting gonadotropin-releasing hormone analogs (leuprolide acetate, cetrorelix) and peripherally acting agents to include aromatase inhibitors, antiprogestins, and selective progesterone receptor modulators (SPRMs). Taken together, the management of leiomyoma depends on given patient's symptoms, age, and desire for future fertility. In the case of women suffering from abnormal uterine bleeding, heavy menstrual bleeding, medical management

With NSAIDs, progestin, combination of oral contraceptives, a levonorgestrel re leasing intrauterine device, or tranexamic acid has been shown to be beneficial.

This manuscript will review the diagnoses, management and treatment of uterine fibroids.

Saverio Danese

In: Uterine Fibroids … ISBN: 978-1-53619-184-4
Editors: Marco Mitidieri et al. © 2021 Nova Science Publishers, Inc.

Chapter 1

IMAGING FEATURES OF MYOMETRIUM AND UTERINE MASSES

Silvia Gemmiti[1,*], MD, Houssein El Hajj[2], MD,
Chiara Benedetto[1], PhD,
Stephanie Anne Sophie Gentile[3], MD
and Donatella Tota[3], MD

[1]Obstetrics and Gynecology 1U, Department of Surgical Sciences,
Sant'Anna Hospital, University of Turin, Turin, Italy
[2]Department of Gynecology and Obstetrics, North West Hospital,
Villefranche-sur-Saône, Gleizé, France
[3]Radiology, Department of Diagnostic Imaging and Radiotherapy,
City of Health and Science, University of Turin, Turin, Italy

ABSTRACT

Uterine leiomyomas are the most common gynaecological tumours and occur in about 20-50% of women around the world. Leiomyomas are

---

[*] Corresponding Author's E-mail: silvia.gemmiti@gmail.com.

the most frequent benign tumours, with an estimated 0.1-0.8% risk of malignant transformation into sarcomas. However malignant leiomyosarcomas are rare and can arise de novo. Ultrasonography is the first line imaging examination in the suspicion of fibroids, as a high sensitivity and specificity test, confirming the existence of fibroids, allowing the differentiation of myomas with adenomyosis, polyps, ovarian tumours, and pregnant uterus. Ultrasound scans can be performed transvaginally or transabdominally; but, in general, transvaginal sonography is superior in most cases. Magnetic resonance imagining provides additional information as a means of further diagnostics in patients in whom ultrasound findings are confusing. MRI is helpful in delineating the anatomy, extent of growth in both benign and malignant diseases, staging of common and uncommon primary uterine malignancies.

INTRODUCTION

Uterine leiomyomas or uterine fibroids are the most common gynaecological tumours and occur in about 20-50% of women around the world, with the highest frequency in groups of black women of reproductive age. As tumours responsive to hormones are rare in prepubertal age, they accelerate in growth during pregnancy and involute with the onset of menopause. Leiomyomas are the most frequent benign tumours, with an estimated 0.1-0.8% risk of malignant transformation into sarcomas.

However malignant leiomyosarcomas are rare and can arise de novo, without leiomyoma as a "base." In the human body, they are the most common tumour of all pelvic organs. Ultrasonography (USG) is the first line imaging examination in the suspicion of fibroids, as a high sensitivity and specificity test. Ultrasound scans can be performed transvaginally (transvaginal scan - TVS) or transabdominally (transabdominal scan - TAS); both scans have advantages and limitations, but, in general, transvaginal sonography is superior to transabdominal sonography in most cases of pelvic pathology. TVS is preferred generally, allowing for detailed assessment of the myometrium within a limited depth of view, is more sensitive in the detection of small leiomyomas and is more useful in cases of retroverted and/or retroflexed uteruses. Moreover, TVS is helpful in patients with large amounts of bowel gas, in those unable to achieve adequate bladder filling, and in obese patients, where TAS is very difficult to perform. TAS was found to be superior in the diagnosis of fundal myomas; nevertheless, TVS is helpful in further assessment of such pathologies. Examination by TVS commences with a dynamic two-dimensional (2D) scan of the uterus in two perpendicular planes. Some gentle pressure applied by either the probe or the examiner's free hand may be required to assess uterine mobility and to screen for site-specific tenderness. TAS may be necessary for imaging beyond the small pelvis. For adequate visualization of the uterus, some bladder filling will be required to displace the small bowel from the field of view. Image quality during TAS may be hampered by adiposity, scar tissue or uterine retroversion. The biggest limitation of TVS is the shallow depth of the scan, thus large or pedunculated myomas may be out of the scan in high frequency probes with short focal lengths. A very important fact is that both TVS as well as TAS are totally operator-dependent types of examination, so their efficiency always depends on the knowledge and skills of the operator.

During ultrasound examination leiomyomas usually appear as well-defined, solid, concentric, hypoechoic masses that cause a variable amount of acoustic shadowing. However, depending on the level of calcification or/and the amount of fibrous tissue, leiomyomas may present different echogenicity, usually hyperechogenic or isoechogenic. Calcifications are seen as echogenic foci with shadowing. Sometimes leiomyomas may have anechogenic components as a result of progressing necrosis. In some difficult cases when leiomyomas are small and isoechogenic to the myometrium, the only visible ultrasound sign may be a bulge in the uterine contour. Leiomyomas of lower uterine segments like the cervix may obstruct the uterine canal.

Consequently, the accumulation of fluid in the endometrial canal might be easy to notice during the examination.

Myometrial pathology may be localized (one or more lesion) or diffuse. A myometrial lesion may be well-defined, as seen typically in fibroids, or ill-defined, as seen typically in adenomyosis. According to MUSA terms each lesion should be described according to its location, size and site. However this is not possible for some ill-defined lesions.

The site of a well-defined lesion should be reported using the FIGO classification for fibroids: 0 = pedunculated intracavitary; 1 = submucosal, <50% intramural; 2 = submucosal, ≥50% intramural; 3 = 100% intramual, but in contact with the endometrium; 4 = intramural; 5 = subserosal, ≥50% intramural; 6 = subserosal, <50% intramural; 7 = subserosal pedunculated; 8 = other (e.g., cervical, parasitic) (Figure 3). Lesion size is estimated by measuring the three largest orthogonal diameters. The minimum distance from the lesion to the endometrium (inner lesion-free margin) and to the serosal surface (outer lesion-free margin) of the uterus is measured. The echogenicity of a lesion is reported as uniform (homogeneous and/or having symmetrical pattern of echogenicity) or non-uniform (heterogeneous) and a uniform lesion may be hypo-, iso- or hyperechogenic. A lesion may have non-uniform echogenicity due to mixed echogenicity or the presence of echogenic areas or cystic areas (regular or irregular). If present, cystic contents may be anechoic, of low-level echogenicity, of ground-glass appearance or of mixed echogenicity.

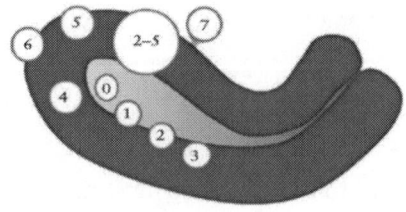

Figure 1. The FIGO classification of myomas (adapted from Munro et al.).

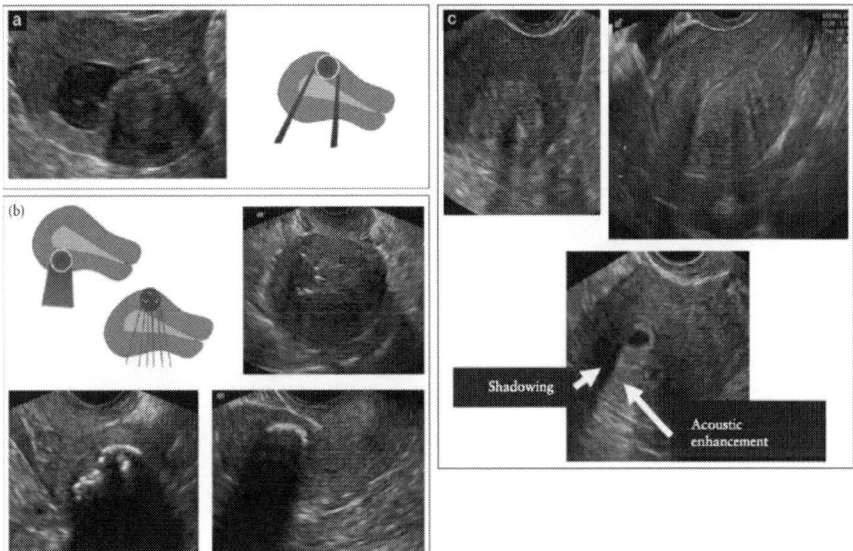

Figure 2. Schematic diagrams and ultrasound images illustrating edge shadowing (a), internal shadowing (b) and fan-shaped shadowing (c). The lower image in (c) also shows an anechogenic myometrial cyst with a hyperechogenic rim surrounding the cyst and acoustic enhancement posterior to the cyst.

Shadowing may arise from the edge of a lesion or from areas within the lesion, they appear as hypoechogenic linear stripes, sometimes alternating with linear hyperechogenic stripes. This type of shadowing may be caused by overlying (micro)cystic structure(s). The degree of shadowing is recorded subjectively as slight, moderate or strong.

The vascular pattern within the myometrium may be uniform or non-uniform and the vascular pattern of a myometrial lesion may be circumferential, intralesional or both.

Some lesions are associated with disruption of the normal uterine vasculature, while others are not. The degree of vascularization should be reported using a subjective color score, the amount of color within a lesion is reported using the color score (1 = no color; 2 = minimal color; 3 = moderate color; 4 = abundant color) (Table 1).

Table 1. Reporting vascularity of the myometrium on ultrasound examination

Vascularization to be assessed	Description	Measurement
Whole uterus		
Overall vessel pattern* (Figure 8)	Uniform, non-uniform*	—
Lesions		
Amount of color (in a lesion)* (Figure S10)	Color score (both percentage of lesion being vascularized and color hue are taken into account)*	No color (1); minimal color (2); moderate color (3); abundant color (4)*
In case of uneven spread of vascularization†	Color score in most vascularized part†	No color (1); minimal color (2); moderate color (3); abundant color (4)†
	Percent of solid tissue with color signal†	0–100%†
	Compared to adjacent myometrium†	Iso-, hypo-, hypervascularity†
Location of vessels† (Figures 8 and 9)	Circumferential, intralesional; uniform, non-uniform (areas with increased/decreased vascularity)†	—
Vessel morphology† (Figures 8 and S11)	Number: single, multiple; size: large and equal, small and equal, unequal; branching: regular, irregular, no branching; direction: perpendicular, not perpendicular†	—

ULTRASOUND FINDINGS ASSOCIATED WITH PATHOLOGY

Fibroid (Leiomyoma)

A uterine fibroid is seen typically on ultrasound as a well-defined round lesion within the myometrium or attached to it, often showing shadows at the edge of the lesion and/or internal fan-shaped shadowing. The echogenicity varies and some hyperechogenicity may be present internally. On color- or power-Doppler Imaging, circumferential flow around the lesion is often visible. However, some fibroids do not exhibit such typical features. We suggest that such fibroids are labelled as sonographically atypical fibroids. On histological examination, fibroids are composed of smooth muscle cells and connective tissue in densely packed whorls. Acoustic shadowing may arise from the interface between smooth muscle bundles, hyalinized connective tissue and normal myometrium. The sonographic appearance of a fibroid may depend on the proportion of muscle cells and fibrous stroma within the lesion.

Uterine Sarcomas and Other Uterine Smooth-Muscle Tumors

Malignant sarcomas comprise leiomyosarcoma, endometrial stromal sarcoma, adenosarcoma and undifferentiated sarcoma. Uterine sarcomas are typically single, large tumors. Their ultrasound features may be indistinct from those of ordinary fibroids or they may appear as an irregularly vascularized mass, with a regular or irregular outline, often with irregular anechoic areas due to necrosis. There are no specific ultrasound features described for Uterine smooth-muscle tumor of uncertain malignant potential (STUMP).

Adenomyosis

Adenomyosis is a difficult to diagnose pathology, due to the lack of significant pathognomonic signs and clinical findings, as well as differences in the histological criteria of adenomyosis recognition. Therefore, intramural leiomyomas are often misdiagnosed as adenomyosis and vice versa. However, some ultrasound features may be helpful in establishing the proper diagnosis. The following findings are suggestive of adenomyosis:

- globular uterine enlargement without the presence of leiomyomata;
- cystic anechoic spaces or lakes in the myometrium;
- subendometrial echoic linear striations;
- uterine wall thickening;
- heterogeneous echo texture;
- obscured endometrial/myometrial border;
- thickening of the transition zone.

Subserosal fibroids and adnexal masses are pathologies that may be very difficult to distinguish. Sometimes subserosal fibroids can be pedunculated or predominantly extrauterine. As a consequence, on ultrasound they might look similar to ovarian tumours. Because of the large fibrous component, ovarian Brenner tumours and fibrothecomas might show a low signal on T2W scans, and sometimes the proper diagnosis is not made until surgery. Another very useful tool in the diagnosis of leiomyomas is colour Doppler ultrasonography. This technique shows circumferential vascularity, blood flow, and arterial supply of the fibroid. Nevertheless, necrotic leiomyomas or those that undergo torsion do not present any blood flow.

Intrauterine benign masses, such as endometrial polyps and submucosal fibroids, are sometimes misdiagnosed, which may result in improper treatment and possible harm to the patient. Multiple, circular feeding vessels are characteristic for fibroids, whereas a single feeding artery can be observed in most polyps. Strain elastography complements sonography in the assessment of intrauterine lesions. Strain elastography may be used to visualise the different stiffness of endometrial polyps and submucosal leiomyomas. Additionally, hysterosonography might be an important addition to TVS in accurate delineation of submucosal and intracavitary leiomyomas. For further diagnostics a 3D TVS may be combined with saline instillation into the uterine cavity to differentiate submucosal leiomyomas and endometrial polyps. Three-dimensional saline contrast sonohysterography may provide even more in-formation in this aspect.

In some cases, magnetic resonance imagining (MRI) provides additional information as a means of further diagnostics in patients in whom ultrasound findings are confusing. With a specificity of 100%, accuracy of 97% and sensitivity in the range 86-92%, it is a great ally in the diagnosis of leiomyomas. Additionally, MRI is helpful in the assessment of the anatomy of the uterus and ovaries as well as in planning of myomectomy. In T1 and T2 MRI scans, leiomyomas appear as areas of low or intermediate signal with sharps margins.

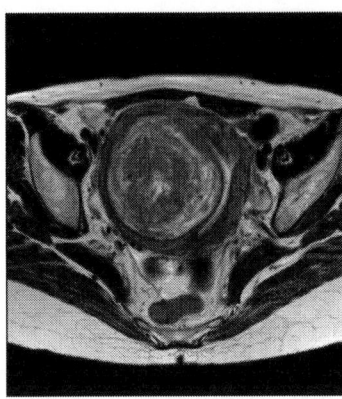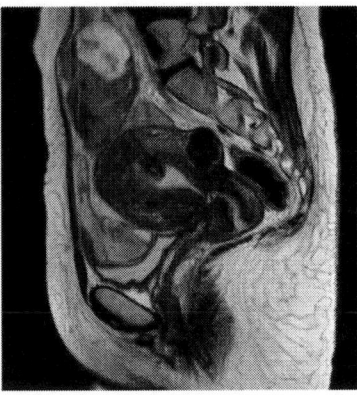

Figure 3. a) Axial T2W MRI shows a large intramural fibroid with internal high signal pressing the endometrial cavity. b) Sagittal T2W MRI image shows multiple fibroid: the largest subserosal lying on the posterior uterine wall; the smallest is intramural. These show typical low-signal intensity.

The most common MRI appearance is a large infiltrating myometrial mass with irregular, ill-defined margins; heterogeneous T1 signal; intermediate- to high-intensity T2 signal and heterogeneous enhancement owing to areas of necrosis and hemorrhage. These characteristics do not differentiate it from benign degenerating fibroids. Rapid growth remains suspicious for leiomyosarcoma though not reliable. In a large retrospective study, less than 3% of leiomyosarcomas, showed rapid growth and leiomyosarcoma was discovered in just 1 woman among 371 women with rapidly growing masses (presumed fibroids). Restricted diffusion and T2 signal of the mass have shown potential for differentiating benign from malignant tumors. These tumors involve the myometrium and have a tendency for lymphatic and vascular invasion, appearing as worm-like bands of low-intensity T2 signal within areas of myometrial involvement.

Dynamic or functional MRI scans improve diagnosis over T2-weighted imaging alone. The addition of gadolinium contrast can highlight the increased vascularity of normal leiomyoma relative to myometrium; however, this is not universal as lack of enhancement may indicate complete degeneration of a benign leiomyoma.

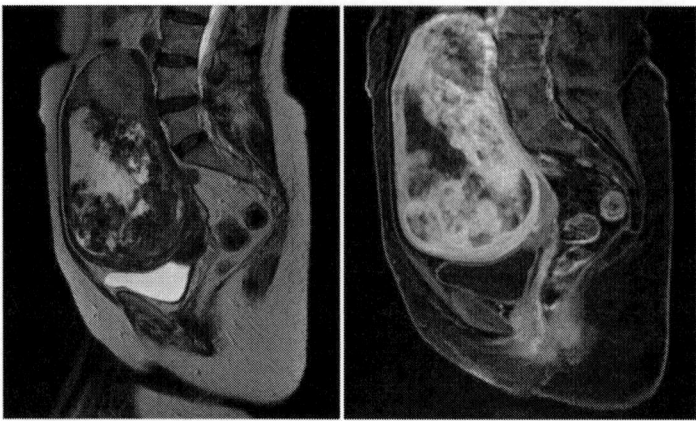

Figure 4. Sagittal T2-weighted MR image (a) shows large lobulated endouterine mass with cystic component. Sagittal contrast-enhancement fat-suppressed T1-weighted MR image (b) demonstrates an heterogeneous high intensity signal arising and protruding into the uterine cavity, causing marked enlargement of the uterus.

Enhancement of lesions at 60 seconds using gadolinium contrast is highly predictive of normal leiomyomata.

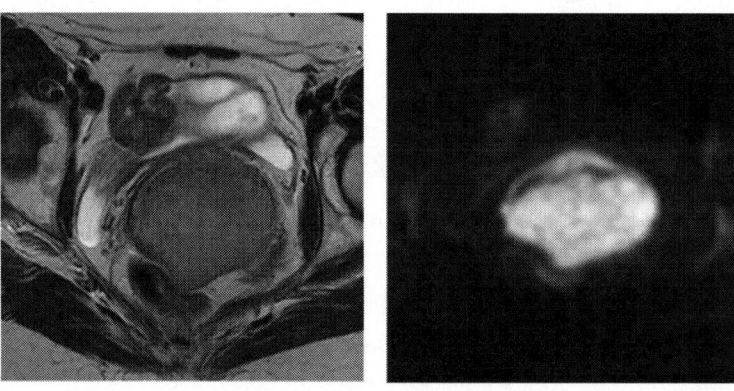

Figure 5. Axial T2W MRI image (a) shows a mass lesion with mildly hyperintense signal. It also shows restricted diffusion on axial DWI high-value (b = 800s/mm²) image (b), with increased signal intensity and corresponding decreased signal intensity seen on ADC map (not shown) raised concern for leiomyosarcoma, which was proven at hysterectomy.

An emerging MRI technique that is widely available and can potentially help distinguish tumors with malignant potential from benign leiomyomas is diffusion weighted imaging (DWI). DWI relies on diffusion motion of water molecules in the extracellular space that is restricted in tumors with high cellularity, such as tumors with malignant potential. DWI can be quantified using an apparent diffusion coefficient (ADC) and used as an adjunct to traditional MRI, but T2- and T1-weighted imaging is still needed to characterize leiomyoma biology.

For instance, leiomyosarcomas tend to have a low ADC, but ADC values overlap with "ordinary" leiomyomas because some ordinary leiomyomas have high ECM content of leiomyomas limiting diffusion. However, a low signal intensity on T2- and T1-weighted imaging and a smooth border would indicate a typical homogeneous, highly fibrotic leiomyoma, even if ADC was low. High signal intensity on T2- and/or T1-weighted images could indicate a leiomyosarcoma, cellular leiomyoma or a degenerated leiomyoma; here, DWI with high ADC may be reassuring that it is morelikely a degenerated leiomyoma while low ADC would be more worrisome but not confirmatory, for malignancy. When ADC and T2-weighted imaging were used together, accuracy for the classification of benign and malignant tumors was 92.4%. Ongoing studies continue to try to improve positive predictive value for malignancy.

CONCLUSION

A wide spectrum of benign and malignant pathologies occur in the uterus. Ultrasound examination is the basic imaging test confirming the existence of fibroids, allowing the differentiation of myomas with adenomyosis, polyps, ovarian tumours, and pregnant uterus. MRI is helpful in delineating the anatomy, extent of growth in both benign and malignant diseases, staging of common and uncommon primary uterine malignancies and response to targeted and systemic treatment.

REFERENCES

[1] Munro M. G., Critchley H. O., Fraser I. S. The FIGO classification of causes of abnormal uterine bleeding in the reproductive years. *Fertil Steril* 2011; 95: 2204-2208.

[2] Matteson K. A., Raker C. A., Clark M. A., Frick K. D. Abnormal uterine bleeding, health status, and usual source of medical care: Analyses using the Medical Expenditures Panel Survey. *J Womens Health* (Larchmt). 2013; 22:959-965.

[3] Van den Bosch T., M. Dueholm, F. P. Leone, et al., Terms, definitions and measurements to describe sonographic features of myometrium and uterine masses: a consensus opinion from the Morphological Uterus Sonographic Assessment (MUSA) group. *Ultrasound Obstet Gynecol*, 46 (2015), pp. 284-298.

[4] Munro M. G., Critchley H. O., Broder M. S., Fraser I. S. FIGO classification system (PALM-COEIN) for causes of abnormal uterine bleeding in nongravid women of reproductive age. *Int J Gynaecol Obstet* 2011; 113: 3-13.

[5] Gordts S., Brosens J. J., Fusi L., Benagiano G., Brosens I. Uterine adenomyosis: a need for uniform terminology and consensus classification. *Reprod Biomed Online* 2008; 17: 244-248.

[6] Hampton T. Critics of fibroid removal procedure question risks it may pose for women with undetected uterine cancer. *JAMA* 2014; 311: 891-893.

[7] Exacoustos C., Brienza L., Di G. A., Szabolcs B., Romanini M. E., Zupi E., Arduini D. Adenomyosis: three-dimensional sonographic findings of the junctional zone and correlation with histology. *Ultrasound Obstet Gynecol* 2011; 37: 471-479.

[8] Martins W. P., Raine-Fenning N. J., Leite S. P., Ferriani R. A., Nastri C. O. A standardized measurement technique may improve the reliability of measurements of endometrial thickness and volume. *Ultrasound Obstet Gynecol* 2011; 38: 107-115.

[9] Abuhamad A. Z., Singleton S., Zhao Y., Bocca S. The Z technique: an easy approach to the display of the mid-coronal plane of the uterus in volume sonography. *J Ultrasound Med* 2006; 25: 607-612.

[10] Wamsteker K., Emanuel M. H., de Kruif J. H. Transcervical hysteroscopic resection of submucous fibroids for abnormal uterine bleeding: results regarding the degree of intramural extension. *Obstet Gynecol* 1993; 82: 736-740.

[11] Casadio P., Youssef A. M., Spagnolo E., Rizzo M. A., Talamo M. R., De A. D., Marra E., Ghi T., Savelli L., Farina A., Pelusi G., Mazzon I. Should the myometrial free margin still be considered a limiting factor for hysteroscopic resection of submucous fibroids? A possible answer to an old question. *Fertil Steril* 2011; 95: 1764-1768.

[12] Timmerman D., Valentin L., Bourne T. H., Collins W. P., Verrelst H., Vergote I. Terms, definitions and measurements to describe the sonographic features of adnexal tumors: a consensus opinion from the International Ovarian Tumor Analysis (IOTA) Group. *Ultrasound Obstet Gynecol* 2000; 16: 500-505.

[13] Alcazar J. L. Three-dimensional power Doppler derived vascular indices: what are we measuring and how are we doing it? *Ultrasound Obstet Gynecol* 2008; 32: 485-487.

[14] Raine-Fenning N. J., Campbell B. K., Clewes J. S., Kendall N. R., Johnson I. R. The reliability of virtual organ computer-aided analysis (VOCAL) for the semiquantification of ovarian, endometrial and subendometrial perfusion. *Ultrasound Obstet Gynecol* 2003; 22: 633-636.

[15] Kishi Y., Suginami H., Kuramori R., Yabuta M., Suginami R., Taniguchi F. Four subtypes of adenomyosis assessed by magnetic

resonance imaging and their specification. *Am J Obstet Gynecol* 2012; 207: 114-117.

[16] Kliewer M. A., Hertzberg B. S., George P. Y., McDonald J. W., Bowie J. D., Carroll B. A. Acoustic shadowing from uterine leiomyomas: sonographic-pathologic correlation. *Radiology* 1995; 196: 99-102.

[17] McLucas B. Diagnosis, imaging and anatomical classification of uterine fibroids. *Best Pract Res Clin Obstet Gynaecol* 2008; 22: 627-642.

[18] Ueda H., Togashi K., Konishi I., Kataoka M. L., Koyama T., Fujiwara T., Kobayashi H., Fujii S., Konishi J. Unusual appearances of uterine leiomyomas: MR imaging findings and their histopathologic backgrounds. *Radiographics* 1999; 19: 131-145.

[19] Karpathiou G., Sivridis E., Giatromanolaki A. Myxoid leiomyosarcoma of the uterus: a diagnostic challenge. *Eur J Gynaecol Oncol* 2010; 31: 446-448.

[20] Bonneau C., Thomassin-Naggara I., Dechoux S., Cortez A., Darai E., Rouzier R. Value of ultrasonography and magnetic resonance imaging for the characterization of uterine mesenchymal tumors. *Acta Obstet Gynecol Scand* 2013; 93: 261-268.

[21] Can gray-scale and color Doppler sonography differentiate between uterine leiomyosarcoma and leiomyoma? *J Clin Ultrasound* 2007; 35: 449-457.

[22] Aviram R., Ochshorn Y., Markovitch O., Fishman A., Cohen I., Altaras M. M., Tepper R. Uterine sarcomas versus leiomyomas: gray-scale and Doppler sonographic findings. *J Clin Ultrasound* 2005; 33: 10-13.

[23] Amant F., Coosemans A., Debiec-Rychter M., Timmerman D., Vergote I. Clinical management of uterine sarcomas. *Lancet Oncol* 2009; 10: 1188-1198.

[24] Vaquero M. E., Magrina J. F., Leslie K. O. Uterine smooth-muscle tumors with unusual growth patterns. *J Minim Invasive Gynecol* 2009; 16: 263-268.

In: Uterine Fibroids ... ISBN: 978-1-53619-184-4
Editors: Marco Mitidieri et al. © 2021 Nova Science Publishers, Inc.

Chapter 2

IMPACT, MANAGEMENT, AND TREATMENT OF UTERINE MYOMAS IN INFERTILE COUPLES

Andrea Carosso*, MD, Alessandro Ruffa, MD, Noemi Mercaldo, MD, Bernadette Evangelisti, MD and Alberto Revelli, PhD

Gynecology and Obstetrics 1U, Pathophysiology of Reproduction and IVF Unit, Department of Surgical Sciences, Sant Anna Hospital, University of Torino, Turin, Italy

ABSTRACT

Uterine myomas (also known as leiomyomas or fibroids) are the most common benign tumors of the female genital tract, occurring in 50-80% of women in reproductive age. The presence of uterine myomas is reported in up to 10% of infertile women, but when all other causes of infertility have been excluded, myomas are found only in 2–3% of cases.

---

* Corresponding Author's E-mail: andrea88.carosso@gmail.com.

Careful diagnostic workup should aim to rule out other possible causes of infertility, with particular attention to the patient's age and ovarian reserve. The clinical management of myomas depends on the number, size, and location. Submucous myomas can considerably distort the uterine cavity and reduce endometrial receptivity and implantation rates, whereas subserous myomas do not appear to affect reproductive outcomes or the risk of spontaneous abortion. The impact of non-cavity-distorting intramural myomas is more controversial and it is not clear whether fertility or assisted reproductive treatments outcomes may be improved by their removal. So far, endometrial distortion should be considered of pivotal importance when the primary aim of surgical treatment is to improve women's fertility.

PREVALENCE AND RISK FACTORS

Uterine myomas (also known as leiomyomas or fibroids) are the most common benign tumors of the female genital tract, occurring in 50-80% of women in reproductive age [1, 2]. A recent systematic review of epidemiological studies on myoma reported a prevalence range of 4.5-68.6% [3], and evaluated the relative strength of putative risk factors in determining it. The risk of developing a large myoma in reproductive age was found to be two to threefold higher in black women than in white women, probably due to ethnic predisposition [4, 5]. Another risk factor with relevant impact of prevalence is age: women aged 41–50 or 51–60 years are ten times more exposed to the risk of developing a myoma than those aged 21–30 years; the age factor declines beyond the sixth decade, reflecting the protective effect of menopause [3]. The impact of estrogens on myoma development appears in the inverse relationship between age at menarche and number of fibroids, regardless of ethnicity [6]; estrogen exposure might also explain the association between myoma and soybean milk consumption [3].

A positive family history of uterine myomas has been identified as a risk factor, indicating a genetic basis for their pathogenesis [3]. The genetic syndrome is hereditary leiomyomatosis and renal cell carcinoma, an autosomal dominant disease characterized by cutaneous and uterine leiomyomatosis associated with papillary renal cell carcinoma; the gene involved in this syndrome encodes fumarate hydratase, an enzyme that affects tumor suppressor mechanisms. Alteration of multiple genes (e.g., MED12, HMGA2, CYP1A1, CYP1B1), protooncogenes (e.g., p27 and p53), signaling pathways (e.g., PI3K-AKT-MTOR), and epigenetic mechanisms have also been reported to be involved in the onset of myomas. Although leiomyomas are believed to be chromosomally fairly stable, cytogenetic abnormalities detected in 40-50% of cases could be associated with their development and growth. In addition to chromosomal changes, point mutations in key regulatory genes and epigenetic changes induced by microRNAs appear to be involved in myoma formation [7]. Finally, the risk of developing myoma is nearly five-fold higher in women with hypertension than in those with normal blood pressure; the increased risk is linked to smooth muscle cell injury and/or cytokine release [8].

Conversely, smoking appears to be a protective factor, at least in women with low body-mass index (BMI, weight in kg divided by the height in square meters), which may result from the putative anti-estrogenic effect of smoking. Parity has also been found to reduce the risk of developing myomas [3]. The association between oral contraceptives and myomas is debated: studies have shown a higher or equal or lower incidence of fibroids among users of combined oral contraceptives [9].

LOCALIZATION

Myomas may arise in different sites. The International Federation of Gynecology and Obstetrics (FIGO) classification system [10] distinguishes eight different localization sites of myomas. Pedunculated intracavitary lesions attached to the endometrium by a narrow stalk are classified as type 0. Submucous leiomyomas with an intramural portion are classified as type 1 or 2, with type 1 being < 50% in mean diameter intramural and type 2 being at least 50% intramural. Type 3 lesions are totally intramural but "touch" the endometrium. Type 4 lesions are intramural leiomyomas arising entirely within the myometrium, without distorting the endometrial cavity and not extending to the serosa. Subserous leiomyomas are categorized in type 5 (at least 50% intramural), type 6 (< 50% intramural), and type 7 (subserous pedunculated). Transmural leiomyomas are in contact with both the endometrial and the serosal surfaces and are classified as type 2–5. Type 8 includes other leiomyomas with no relation to the myometrium (e.g., those within the broad ligament).

DIAGNOSIS

The diagnostic workup of uterine myomas includes ultrasound examination, hysteroscopy, sono-hysterography, and magnetic resonance imaging (MRI).

Ultrasound is widely used as the first tool for detecting and evaluating myometrial alterations: it is easy to perform, accessible, safe, and cost-effective. It provides an accurate assessment of myoma diameter, echogenicity, and location [11]. For better clarity, ultrasonographic features should be described and reported using the MUSA (Morphological Uterus Sonographic Assessment) terminology [12].

Transvaginal ultrasonography (TV-US) provides detailed image resolution, as the probe is positioned in close proximity to the uterus and allows a more precise view of the endometrium than the transabdominal approach. Though TV-US imaging is not constrained by obesity, bowel gas or retroverted uterus [13], transabdominal ultrasound is more effective than TV-US for evaluating subserous myomas extending into the abdominal cavity [11] and very large myomas [14]. Transvaginal and transabdominal US can be easily combined and are widely used together for detecting, mapping, measuring, and characterizing myomas [11]. However, ultrasound may be not sufficient to assess multiple myomas and to accurately describe distortion of the endometrial cavity. Preoperative assessment of submucous myomas (FIGO 0-2) should include evaluation of the degree of endometrial involvement; therefore, the addition of hysteroscopy or sono-hysterography is recommended [14].

Sono-hysterography (US examination with simultaneous infusion of saline as contrast medium into the uterine cavity) is a simple and well-tolerated procedure, with the same accuracy as hysteroscopy in assessing submucous myoma location, extent of attachment, and intracavitary protrusion [11]. Sono-hysterography and diagnostic hysteroscopy can also be considered complementary methods before hysteroscopic myomectomy [15]. Three-dimensional (3D) US may be a useful tool to reconstruct the coronal plane of the uterus, which usually cannot be visualized by traditional 2-dimensional (2D) imaging [16, 17]; it has high diagnostic accuracy and high specificity in detecting uterine cavity abnormalities (e.g., submucous myomas) but its sensitivity is limited, particularly in the detection of endometrial polyps and in the differential diagnosis with FIGO 0-1 myomas.

Currently, hysteroscopy is still considered the gold standard for the investigation of the uterine cavity [18]. Type 3 myomas can be clearly distinguished from type 2 myomas only by hysteroscopy: the intrauterine inflation pressure should be kept as low as possible to allow for correct visualization of the endometrial cavity and of the relationships between myoma, endometrium, and myometrium. In this way, misdiagnosis of a submucous myoma as a type 3 myoma can be avoided [10].

MRI is the most accurate and reliable imaging technique for myoma mapping and characterization by virtue of its high tissue contrast resolution and reproducibility. Since it is by far less accessible and more expensive than US, it should be reserved for selected cases. Indications for MRI in the diagnostic workup include the differential diagnosis with adenomyosis, smooth muscle tumor with uncertain malignant potential (STUMP,) and malignant leiomyosarcoma [11].

REPRODUCTIVE OUTCOME

Uterine myoma is reported in up to 10% of infertile women, but only 2–3% of cases of infertility may be attributed to the myoma after all other causes have been excluded [19]. With the shift of childbearing to the fourth and fifth decades of life, the detection of myomas in women seeking pregnancy is likely to become ever more common in the near future.

Globally, the presence of an uterine myoma is associated with lower chance of spontaneous and medically-assisted conception [20]. Several mechanisms by which a myoma may adversely affect fertility have been hypothesized [19]. Recent evidence suggests that myomas may impair fertility by interfering with endometrial receptivity and embryo implantation. Molecular studies have demonstrated that homeobox (HOX) gene expression is one of the complex molecular events involved in endometrial receptivity and that their down-regulation results in defective decidualization, which may hinder implantation [21]. HOXA-10 is regulated by bone morphogenetic protein 2 (BMP-2), a growth factor inhibited by transforming growth factor-β3 (TGF-β3) [22]. Myomas are thought to be responsible for the overexpression of TGF-b3; HOXA-10 levels are consequently reduced in the endometrium of women with myomas, in both the part of the endometrium overlying the leiomyoma and throughout the endometrial cavity [23]. Altered vascularization and chronic endometrial inflammation are other hypothetical mechanisms implicated in impaired fertility: myomas induce higher local levels of monocyte chemoattractant protein-1 (MCP-1), leading to accumulation of macrophages, synthesis of PGF2α, and local inflammatory status [24]. Other possible explanations for the detrimental effects of myoma on reproductive outcomes are the anatomic distortion of the uterine cavity and the increased or abnormal myometrial contractility, which may interfere with sperm migration, embryo transport and implantation. Overall, the effect of myoma on fertility is largely related to its location, size, and number. Current evidence suggests that myoma location plays a prominent role in fertility and pregnancy outcome: submucous myomas exert the worse adverse effect on reproductive outcomes, whereas subserous myomas do not appear to affect fertility or the risk of spontaneous abortion [20, 25]. Compared to infertile women without myomas, women with submucous myomas undergoing medically assisted reproduction (MAR) have a significantly lower pregnancy rate, implantation rate, and live birth rate, and a much higher spontaneous abortion rate [20].

While submucous myomas always distort the uterine cavity and subserous myomas never do, intramural myomas can be either distorting or non-distorting: intramural myomas that distort the uterine cavity seem to have a negative impact on MAR efficacy [20]. Differently, the impact of non-cavity-distorting intramural myomas is controversial and it is not clear whether fertility may be improved by their removal [20, 26, 27]. Two systematic reviews reported a 21-44% reduction in live birth rate and a 15-32% reduction in clinical pregnancy rate in women with non-cavity-distorting intramural myomas undergoing IVF compared to women without myoma [27, 28]. Though not statistically significant, the implantation rate was lower and the miscarriage rate higher in these patients. Both studies indicated that non-cavity-distorting intramural myoma may have a negative impact on IVF success [27, 28].

Distinguishing between type 3, 4, and 5 myomas may be important because of the impact on fertility: a type 3 myoma may impact more on implantation because of its contact with the endometrium, resulting in impaired decidualization [29]. A study investigating the impact of type 3 intramural myomas on IVF outcome reported a negative effect only when the size of the myoma was at least 2 cm in diameter [29].

The lower live birth rate after IVF in women with non-cavity-distorting intramural myoma does not necessarily mean that myoma removal will restore the live birth rate to the levels expected in women without myoma. Myomectomy can be associated with considerable morbidity, and to date there is insufficient evidence to justify routine intervention in women undergoing IVF and in those trying to conceive naturally [27]. The relative effect of multiple or differently sized myomas on fertility is uncertain [27, 30]. There is inconclusive evidence that large intramural myoma (> 5 cm) has a negative impact on pregnancy and that multiple myomas are a major predictor of spontaneous pregnancy loss [31].

OBSTETRIC OUTCOME

Uterine myomas are relatively common during pregnancy (prevalence, 1.6-10.7%) [32]. A recent study reported that uterine myomas have a distinct growth pattern during pregnancy, with a major increase in size during the first trimester [33]. Between the first and the second trimester, the size increased by 54-75%, likely due to stimulation by sex steroid hormones and human chorionic gonadotrophin (hCG) [34]. After the second trimester, myoma growth slowed to a minimum near the end of gestation; the initial myoma size did not seem to influence its growth pattern during pregnancy. Most women diagnosed with a myoma during pregnancy are asymptomatic and the diagnosis is incidental on US examination for other indications [35].

Myomas have been associated with adverse obstetric outcomes, antepartum and peripartum complications. The relationship between myoma and increased risk of spontaneous abortion remains debated. Two reviews reported an increased risk of miscarriage in women with myomas compared to those without myomas [20, 31]. The mechanisms thought to cause miscarriage are: placental implantation over the myoma, with consequent impaired vascularization and placental insufficiency; myoma degeneration, with release of prostaglandins; distortion of the uterine cavity [36]. Conversely, a recent systematic review and meta-analysis reported no association between myoma and a higher risk of spontaneous abortion in the general obstetric population [37].

Despite the low-moderate quality of published studies, a systematic review of unadjusted cumulative pregnancy outcome in women with myomas [31] reported that uterine myomas are associated with an increased risk of cesarean delivery, largely attributable to fetal malpresentation or dystocia during labor. The risk of preterm labor and preterm birth also appears to be slightly elevated [31]. Myomas > 5 cm, multiple myomas, and placental implantation over a myoma may increase this risk [38]. The mechanisms thought to cause preterm birth are: decreased uterine distensibility with advancing gestation, decreased oxytokinase activity, which may result in higher oxytocin levels within the uterus [39], and chronic inflammation with cytokine release predisposing to premature contractions [40]. Cumulative data suggest that myomas do not increase the risk of premature rupture of membranes [32].

Published studies on placenta abruption in women with myomas have produced contradictory results. While information about uterine myoma size and location is not always clear, myoma is a recognized risk factor for placenta abruption [41] and for placenta previa, likely due to interference or distortion of normal perfusion at the placental site [42].

The most common postpartum complication is hemorrhage, which is likely due to uterine atony [31]. The risk of postpartum hemorrhage (PPH) is higher especially if myomas are > 3 cm in diameter and are located behind the placenta, as well as after cesarean section [32]. Another consequence of altered uterine contractility due to myomas is the increased need for emergency hysterectomy after delivery [31].

Most uterine fibroids tend to decrease in volume after delivery. Only three studies to date have compared myoma size before and after childbirth. A substantial reduction in myoma size during the puerperium has been reported [43] [44], though the evidence is not conclusive [45]. The mechanisms underlying a possible reduction in myoma diameter during the postpartum period are not yet fully understood. Uterine involution seems to play a crucial role: transient uterine ischemia after childbirth is responsible for lesions involving the myoma cells more than the normal myometrium [46]. In addition, breastfeeding seems to be associated with a possible reduction in myoma size during the puerperium: breastfeeding induces a reduction in estrogen and progesterone levels and the exposure to lower steroid concentrations reduces the size of myomas during puerperium. However, Terry et al. reported an inverse association between breastfeeding and the size reduction of fibroids, while Laughlin et al. found no relationship between breastfeeding and a reduction in fibroids [47, 48]. These discrepant results can be explained by the heterogeneity of myoma classification in the study.

TREATMENT

Current strategies in the management of myoma rely mainly on surgical intervention, but the choice of the treatment is ultimately guided by the patient's age and the desire to preserve fertility. Management also depends on the number, size, and location of the myoma. Surgical and non-surgical approaches include myomectomy by hysteroscopy, myomectomy by laparotomy or laparoscopy, uterine artery embolization and other interventions performed under radiologic or ultrasound guidance to induce thermal ablation of the myoma [15].

SURGICAL TREATMENT

SMM – Submucous Myoma

In couples with unexplained infertility and in those undergoing IVF, hysteroscopic myomectomy is advisable to treat submucous myomas (FIGO 0-2) [14, 20, 49, 50], since the procedure may probably improve IVF results. FIGO 2 myomas are more difficult to resect and may therefore require a two-stage procedure, especially if larger than 3 cm. In patients with infertility it may be preferable to remove large FIGO 2 myomas by laparoscopy, since the onset of endometrial damage and synechiae after multiple hysteroscopic procedures may compromise its function of promoting embryo implantation [51].

The most recent Cochrane meta-analysis found limited evidence for performing myomectomy in infertile women with myomas: no substantial difference in clinical pregnancy rates was found between women who received hysteroscopic myomectomy before IVF and the expectant management group. This finding suggests that myomectomy may not be necessary for improving reproductive outcomes in women with submucous myomas [52].

In light of this evidence, the benefits of myomectomy should be weighed against the risks. Adverse events during hysteroscopic myomectomy are uncommon and include mainly: the intravasation syndrome (OHIA, operative hysteroscopic intravascular absorption) that leads to hyponatremia and blood volume overload (< 1% of cases); uterine perforation; intestinal, vesical, and vascular injuries; intra- and post-operative metrorrhagia; gaseous embolism; infection; intrauterine adhesions. Estrogen therapy is often initiated after operative hysteroscopy to prevent intrauterine adhesions (IUA); however, evidence for the benefit of this approach is scarce and randomized controlled trials are lacking [53]. Early second-look hysteroscopic evaluation after myomectomy is advisable to assess intracavitary outcomes, particularly after multiple myomectomy [50].

IMM – Intramural Myoma

Currently, there is no evidence that myomectomy can improve reproductive outcome in infertile women with intramural myomas; the effectiveness of the procedure remains controversial. The decision whether or not to carry out myomectomy for intramural myomas in a non-distorted endometrial cavity needs to be individualized and should be taken after thorough counseling. The decision may depend on several variables: duration of infertility, woman's age, number and size of the intramural myomas, relationship between the myoma and the uterine cavity, partner's semen parameters, previous pelvic surgery, obstetric history, and history of previous IVF failures. Removal of subserous myomas is not recommended [14].

When myomectomy is indicated, current evidence does not favor any particular surgical approach (laparoscopy, laparotomy, or electrosurgical systems) to improve the rate of live births, preterm delivery, clinical pregnancy, ongoing pregnancy, miscarriage or cesarean section. Furthermore, the evidence needs to be interpreted with caution because of the limited number of studies and the low quality of evidence [52].

The procedure of choice for the best short-term outcome after surgery for a single intramural myoma (diameter ≤ 5 cm) is laparoscopic myomectomy [54, 55]. Compared to mini-laparotomy, laparoscopy is associated with a lower decline in hemoglobin concentration, a reduced length of postoperative ileus, and a shorter time to discharge [56]. In patients with a single large intramural myoma (diameter > 5 cm) or multiple intramural myomas, myomectomy can be performed either laparoscopically or by laparotomic surgery. A valid alternative is mini-laparotomic myomectomy, which offers the same reproductive advantages as laparoscopic surgery, especially in women with unexplained infertility [57]. Major complications of laparoscopic myomectomy are intraoperative and postoperative hemorrhage requiring blood transfusion and conversion to laparotomy, abdominal-pelvic adhesion formation, and IUA [58]. Need for conversion to hysterectomy to control hemorrhage during abdominal myomectomy has been reported in 2% of cases [59].

Open myomectomy was compared to laparoscopic myomectomy in two randomized clinical trials: no significant difference was noted for miscarriage rate, preterm labor rate, and cesarean section rate [26]. There were no significant differences between the two groups in perinatal outcome: rate of emergency cesarean section, preterm delivery, placental abnormality, pregnancy-induced hypertension, low Apgar score, non-reassuring fetal heart pattern, intrauterine fetal death, and incidence of PPH [60].

Uterine rupture during pregnancy and labor is one of the most severe long-term complications after myomectomy. Risk factors for uterine rupture are opening of the uterine cavity, electrocoagulation, single-layer suture, hematoma formation [61], and the time interval between myomectomy and pregnancy [62]. In the absence of hematoma or myometrial edema after myomectomy, the scarred uterus recovers its anatomical stability in about 12 weeks after myomectomy. To reduce the risk of uterine rupture, patients should wait at least 3-6 months after myomectomy before seeking pregnancy [63]. A longer time interval between myomectomy and conception may have a detrimental effect on reproductive outcome, however, especially in women of late reproductive age. Embryo cryopreservation before myomectomy may be an effective approach in patients of advanced age, with poor ovarian reserve and cavity-distorting myomas. Although a common strategy, its efficacy has not yet been widely evaluated [64]. The overall incidence of uterine rupture after myomectomy is 0.93% during pregnancy and labor [65]. Given the low incidence, trial of labor after myomectomy may be considered and offered as a feasible and relatively safe option [66].

Recent developments in surgical techniques for myomectomy include robotic surgery and gasless laparoscopic myomectomy (GLM). GLM seems to be more feasible, safer, and more effective than other minimally invasive techniques in reducing blood loss, postoperative abdominal pain, and recurrence rate. More evidence is needed to determine its long-term effects via adequate studies investigating the value of GLM in more complicated cases [67].

Robotic approaches offer the advantages of three dimensional visualization, greater dexterity, no hand tremor, and less surgeon fatigue, as well as the benefits of minimally invasive techniques such as less blood loss, less need for blood transfusion, and shorter hospital stay [68]. A prospective non-randomized cohort study noted that both laparoscopic and robotic myomectomy reduce the severity of symptoms associated with fibroids and improve the quality of life at 1 year after surgery. However, the costs related to robotic surgery still limit its wider application [69].

Laparoscopic ligature of the uterine artery, laparoscopic cryo-myolysis, laparoscopic thermo-coagulation (with monopolar/bipolar current or laser), thermal ablation with laparoscopic or hysteroscopic radio frequency, focused ultrasound surgery under MR guidance (MRgFUS), and uterine artery embolization (UAE) have been proposed as alternative techniques. The limitation common to all these techniques is the lack of histological evaluation of the uterine lesion, which could result in underdiagnosis of malignant tumor [70].

MRgFUS and UAE are contraindicated in women planning future pregnancy [71]. Lower pregnancy rates, higher miscarriage rates, and more adverse pregnancy outcomes have been associated with UAE than with myomectomy [14]. Studies also suggest that UAE is associated with detrimental effects on ovarian reserve, especially in older patients, due to possible anastomosis between uterine and ovarian arteries (46% of women) and subsequent inadvertent embolization of ovarian tissue [51].

MEDICAL THERAPY

Medical therapy for myomas includes administration of gonadotropin-releasing hormone (GnRH) agonists and selective progesterone receptor modulators (SPRMs).

GnRH analogues induce a state of temporary menopause with amenorrhea, suppression of ovulation, and hypoestrogenism. Therapy should not be administered for more than 6 months because of serious side effects (e.g., decreased bone density) [15] and it has no role as stand-alone treatment in infertile women [14]. The advantages of GnRH-analogue therapy are reduction in myoma size, less menstrual bleeding, and improved anemia. A possible complication during myomectomy is the loss of a clear cleavage plane [72].

SPRMs, such as mifepristone, asoprisnil, telapristone acetate, and, notably, ulipristal acetate (UPA), modulate the progesterone pathway which has a crucial role in myoma pathophysiology. Recent research on myoma development and growth has focused on progesterone receptors: Tsigkou et al. reported that PR-B mRNA and PR-A and PR-B proteins are more concentrated in myomas than in the matched myometrium [73]. SPRMs can have an agonistic or antagonist effect on PRs.

There is growing evidence that treatment with UPA prior to IVF treatment may obviate the need for surgery; the pregnancy rate of women treated by UPA was comparable to a control group without myomas [74]. UPA may be an excellent option to reduce myoma size prior to surgery, avoiding the side effects of GnRH-a and ensuring comparable feasibility [75]. Conversely, UPA may require less time to achieve control of bleeding; it maintains a sustained effect (up to 6 months) after completion of treatment compared to the GnRH analogues [71, 76]. UPA is usually administered (daily dose of 5 mg) in treatment protocols of 12 weeks for a maximum of four times with a 2-month mandatory break between cycles [71, 76]. This course of UPA was found to maximize its potential benefits for bleeding control and myoma volume reduction [72]. Long-term intermittent UPA administration is likely to change the approach to the management of uterine myoma. Dolmans and Donnez designed a new therapeutic algorithm: in type 1 FIGO myomas > 3 cm or in patients with anemia, they suggested UPA treatment to reduce myoma size and restore hemoglobin levels. In young infertile women of reproductive age wishing to conceive, with multiple ($\geq$ 2), type 2 or type 2–5 myomas, UPA therapy can be administered in two courses of 3 months each; if the uterine cavity is no longer distorted, the patient can try to conceive naturally or undergo IVF if indicated. If myoma regression is significant ($\geq$ 25%) but the uterine cavity remains distorted or the myoma remains large, surgery is indicated. Response to medical therapy is inadequate in approximately 20% of cases, leaving surgery as the only option. However, UPA may facilitate surgery and allow for a less invasive intervention [71, 76].

Common adverse events associated with UPA therapy include headaches, hot flashes, and breast discomfort; however, they did not lead to a significant dropout rate from treatment [77, 78]. Nonetheless, other serious adverse side effects have been reported. UPA induces the so-called progesterone receptor modulator-associated endometrial changes (PAECs) in almost 70% of patients by the end of treatment. Common adverse side effects are large cystic endometrial glands and changes within the stromal compartment including increased concentration of fibroblasts and vascularization [79]. Such effects on the endometrium are benign and reversible and disappear after two menstrual periods in most cases [71]. Following reports of drug-induced liver injury, including five cases of liver transplantation in patients taking UPA, in March 2020 the European Medicines Agency (EMA) called for temporary discontinuation of UPA therapy until completion of a new drug safety review [80].

The pathogenesis of leiomyoma involves genetic and epigenetic factors, sex steroids, growth factors, chemokines, and extracellular matrix components. A medical therapy that modulates these factors may be useful [81–85]. Among the alternative drugs in the newest therapeutic protocols are epigallocatechin, pirfenidone, and aromatase inhibitors.

A randomized control trial found that an aromatase inhibitor was superior to the GnRH agonist in reducing the total fibroid volume (45.6% vs. 33.2%) [86]. Furthermore, a novel oral SPRM (vilaprisan) [87], orally formulated GnRH receptor antagonists, and a vaginal delivery formulation of GnRH-a (leuprolide) are currently under development for the management of uterine myomas [76].

CONCLUSION

Uterine myomas are a common finding in women presenting with infertility. When all other causes of infertility have been excluded, myomas are found in a few cases. Age may confound the results of studies seeking to clarify the relationship between myoma and infertility. Careful diagnostic workup should rule out other possible causes of infertility, with particular attention to patient age and ovarian reserve.

While there is current evidence that submucous myomas can considerably distort the uterine cavity and reduce endometrial receptivity and implantation rates, data on intramural myomas and their treatment are conflicting. Endometrial distortion should be given pivotal importance in the choice of treatment and should be confirmed by hysteroscopy assessment.

REFERENCES

[1] Baird D D, Dunson D B, Hill M C, Cousins D, Schectman J M. High cumulative incidence of uterine leiomyoma in black and white women: ultrasound evidence. *Am. J. Obstet. Gynecol.* 2003;188:100–7. https://doi.org/10.1067/mob.2003.99.

[2] Cotrino I, Carosso A, Macchi C, Poma C B, Cosma S, Ribotta M, et al. Ultrasound and clinical characteristics of uterine smooth muscle tumors of uncertain malignant potential. *European Journal of Obstetrics & Gynecology and Reproductive Biology* 2020. https://doi.org/10.1016/j.ejogrb.2020.05.040.

[3] Stewart E A, Cookson C L, Gandolfo R A, Schulze-Rath R. Epidemiology of uterine fibroids: a systematic review. *BJOG* 2017;124:1501–12. https://doi.org/10.1111/1471-0528.14640.

[4] Huyck K L, Panhuysen C I M, Cuenco K T, Zhang J, Goldhammer H, Jones E S, et al. The impact of race as a risk factor for symptom severity and age at diagnosis of uterine leiomyomata among affected sisters. *Am. J. Obstet. Gynecol.* 2008;198:168.e1-9. https://doi.org/10.1016/j.ajog.2007.05.038.

[5] Peddada S D, Laughlin S K, Miner K, Guyon J-P, Haneke K, Vahdat H L, et al. Growth of uterine leiomyomata among premenopausal black and white women. *Proc. Natl. Acad. Sci. USA* 2008;105:19887–92. https://doi.org/10.1073/pnas.0808188105.

[6] Velez Edwards D R, Baird D D, Hartmann K E. Association of age at menarche with increasing number of fibroids in a cohort of women who underwent standardized ultrasound assessment. *Am.*

J. Epidemiol. 2013;178:426–33. https://doi.org/10.1093/aje/kws 585.

[7] Pavone D, Clemenza S, Sorbi F, Fambrini M, Petraglia F. Epidemiology and Risk Factors of Uterine Fibroids. *Best Pract Res. Clin. Obstet. Gynaecol.* 2018;46:3–11. https://doi.org/10.1016/j.bpobgyn.2017.09.004.

[8] Boynton-Jarrett R, Rich-Edwards J, Malspeis S, Missmer S A, Wright R. A Prospective Study of Hypertension and Risk of Uterine Leiomyomata. *Am. J. Epidemiol.* 2005;161:628–38. https://doi.org/10.1093/aje/kwi072.

[9] Wise L A, Laughlin-Tommaso S K. Epidemiology of Uterine Fibroids: From Menarche to Menopause. *Clin. Obstet. Gynecol.* 2016;59:2–24. https://doi.org/10.1097/GRF.0000000000000164.

[10] Munro M G, Critchley H O D, Fraser I S, FIGO Menstrual Disorders Committee. The two FIGO systems for normal and abnormal uterine bleeding symptoms and classification of causes of abnormal uterine bleeding in the reproductive years: 2018 revisions. *Int. J. Gynaecol. Obstet.* 2018;143:393–408. https://doi.org/10.1002/ijgo.12666.

[11] Testa A C, Di Legge A, Bonatti M, Manfredi R, Scambia G. Imaging techniques for evaluation of uterine myomas. *Best Pract. Res. Clin. Obstet. Gynaecol.* 2016;34:37–53. https://doi.org/10.1016/j.bpobgyn.2015.11.014.

[12] Van den Bosch T, Dueholm M, Leone F P G, Valentin L, Rasmussen CK, Votino A, et al. Terms, definitions and measurements to describe sonographic features of myometrium and uterine masses: a consensus opinion from the Morphological Uterus Sonographic Assessment (MUSA) group. *Ultrasound Obstet. Gynecol.* 2015;46:284–98. https://doi.org/10.1002/uog.14806.

[13] McLucas B. Diagnosis, imaging and anatomical classification of uterine fibroids. *Best Pract. Res. Clin. Obstet. Gynaecol.* 2008;22:627–42. https://doi.org/10.1016/j.bpobgyn.2008.01.006.

[14] Carranza-Mamane B, Havelock J, Hemmings R, Reproductive Endocrinology and Infertility Committee, Special Contributor. The management of uterine fibroids in women with otherwise unexplained infertility. *J. Obstet. Gynaecol. Can.* 2015;37:277–85. https://doi.org/10. 1016/ S1701-2163(15)30318-2.

[15] Donnez J, Dolmans M-M. Uterine fibroid management: from the present to the future. *Hum. Reprod. Update* 2016;22:665–86. https://doi.org/10.1093/humupd/dmw023.

[16] Andreotti R F, Fleischer A C. Practical applications of 3D sonography in gynecologic imaging. *Radiol. Clin. North Am.* 2014;52:1201–13. https://doi.org/10.1016/j.rcl.2014.07.001.

[17] Wong L, White N, Ramkrishna J, Araujo Júnior E, Meagher S, Costa FDS. Three-dimensional imaging of the uterus: The value of the coronal plane. *World J. Radiol.* 2015;7:484–93. https://doi.org/10.4329/wjr.v7.i12.484.

[18] Apirakviriya C, Rungruxsirivorn T, Phupong V, Wisawasukmongchol W. Diagnostic accuracy of 3D-transvaginal ultrasound in detecting uterine cavity abnormalities in infertile patients as compared with hysteroscopy. *European Journal of Obstetrics and Gynecology and Reproductive Biology* 2016;200: 24–8. https://doi.org/10.1016/j.ejogrb.2016.01.023.

[19] Practice Committee of American Society for Reproductive Medicine in collaboration with Society of Reproductive Surgeons. Myomas and reproductive function. *Fertil. Steril.* 2008;90:S125-130. https://doi.org/10.1016/j.fertnstert.2008.09.012.

[20] Pritts E A, Parker W H, Olive D L. Fibroids and infertility: an updated systematic review of the evidence. *Fertil. Steril.* 2009;91:1215–23. https://doi.org/10.1016/j.fertnstert.2008.01.051.

[21] Munro MG. Uterine polyps, adenomyosis, leiomyomas, and endometrial receptivity. *Fertil. Steril.* 2019;111:629–40. https://doi. org/10.1016/j.fertnstert.2019.02.008.

[22] Doherty L F, Taylor H S. Leiomyoma-derived transforming growth factor-β impairs bone morphogenetic protein-2-mediated

endometrial receptivity. *Fertil. Steril.* 2015;103:845–52. https://doi.org/10.1016/j.fertnstert.2014.12.099.

[23] Rackow B W, Taylor H S. Submucosal uterine leiomyomas have a global effect on molecular determinants of endometrial receptivity. *Fertil. Steril.* 2010;93:2027–34. https://doi.org/10.1016/j.fertnstert.2008.03.029.

[24] Miura S, Khan K N, Kitajima M, Hiraki K, Moriyama S, Masuzaki H, et al. Differential infiltration of macrophages and prostaglandin production by different uterine leiomyomas. *Hum. Reprod.* 2006;21:2545–54. https://doi.org/10.1093/humrep/del 205.

[25] Somigliana E, Vercellini P, Daguati R, Pasin R, De Giorgi O, Crosignani P G. Fibroids and female reproduction: a critical analysis of the evidence. *Hum. Reprod. Update* 2007;13:465–76. https://doi.org/10.1093/humupd/dmm013.

[26] Metwally M, Farquhar C M, Li T C. Is another meta-analysis on the effects of intramural fibroids on reproductive outcomes needed? *Reprod. Biomed.* Online 2011;23:2–14. https://doi.org/10.1016/j.rbmo.2010.08.006.

[27] Sunkara S K, Khairy M, El-Toukhy T, Khalaf Y, Coomarasamy A. The effect of intramural fibroids without uterine cavity involvement on the outcome of IVF treatment: a systematic review and meta-analysis. *Hum. Reprod.* 2010;25:418–29. https://doi.org/10.1093/humrep/dep396.

[28] Rikhraj K, Tan J, Taskin O, Albert A Y, Yong P, Bedaiwy M A. The Impact of Noncavity-Distorting Intramural Fibroids on Live Birth Rate in In Vitro Fertilization Cycles: A Systematic Review and Meta-Analysis. *J. Womens Health* (Larchmt) 2020;29:210–9. https://doi.org/10.1089/jwh.2019.7813.

[29] Yan L, Yu Q, Zhang Y-N, Guo Z, Li Z, Niu J, et al. Effect of type 3 intramural fibroids on in vitro fertilization-intracytoplasmic sperm injection outcomes: a retrospective cohort study. *Fertil.*

Steril. 2018;109:817-822.e2. https://doi.org/10.1016/j.fertnstert. 2018.01.007.

[30] Somigliana E, De Benedictis S, Vercellini P, Nicolosi A E, Benaglia L, Scarduelli C, et al. Fibroids not encroaching the endometrial cavity and IVF success rate: a prospective study. *Hum. Reprod.* 2011;26:834–9. https://doi.org/10.1093/humrep/der015.

[31] Klatsky P C, Tran N D, Caughey A B, Fujimoto V Y. Fibroids and reproductive outcomes: a systematic literature review from conception to delivery. *Am. J. Obstet. Gynecol.* 2008;198:357–66. https://doi.org/10.1016/j.ajog.2007.12.039.

[32] Ezzedine D, Norwitz E R. Are Women With Uterine Fibroids at Increased Risk for Adverse Pregnancy Outcome? *Clin. Obstet. Gynecol.* 2016;59:119–27. https://doi.org/10.1097/GRF.0000000000000169.

[33] Chill H H, Karavani G, Rachmani T, Dior U, Tadmor O, Shushan A. Growth pattern of uterine leiomyoma along pregnancy. *BMC Womens Health* 2019;19:100. https://doi.org/10.1186/s12905-019-0803-5.

[34] Sarais V, Cermisoni G C, Schimberni M, Alteri A, Papaleo E, Somigliana E, et al. Human Chorionic Gonadotrophin as a Possible Mediator of Leiomyoma Growth during Pregnancy: Molecular Mechanisms. *Int. J. Mol. Sci.* 2017;18. https://doi.org/10.3390/ijms18092014.

[35] Gupta S, Jose J, Manyonda I. Clinical presentation of fibroids. *Best. Pract. Res. Clin. Obstet. Gynaecol.* 2008;22:615–26. https://doi.org/10.1016/j.bpobgyn.2008.01.008.

[36] De Vivo A, Mancuso A, Giacobbe A, Savasta L M, De Dominici R, Dugo N, et al. Uterine myomas during pregnancy: a longitudinal sonographic study. *Ultrasound Obstet. Gynecol.* 2011;37:361–5. https://doi.org/10.1002/uog.8826.

[37] Sundermann A C, Velez Edwards D R, Bray M J, Jones S H, Latham S M, Hartmann K E. Leiomyomas in Pregnancy and

Spontaneous Abortion: A Systematic Review and Meta-analysis. *Obstet. Gynecol.* 2017;130:1065–72. https://doi.org/10.1097/AOG.0000000000002313.

[38] Roberts W E, Fulp K S, Morrison J C, Martin J N. The impact of leiomyomas on pregnancy. *Aust. N. Z. J. Obstet. Gynaeco*l. 1999;39:43–7. https://doi.org/10.1111/j.1479-828x.1999.tb0 3442.x.

[39] Blum M. Comparative study of serum CAP activity during pregnancy in malformed and normal uterus. *Journal of Perinatal Medicine* 1978;6:165–8. https://doi.org/10.1515/jpme.1978.6.3.165.

[40] Patterson-Keels L M, Selvaggi S M, Haefner H K, Randolph J F. Morphologic assessment of endometrium overlying submucosal leiomyomas. *J. Reprod. Med.* 1994;39:579–84.

[41] Jenabi E, Zagami S E. The association between uterine leiomyoma and placenta abruption: A meta-analysis. *The Journal of Maternal-Fetal & Neonatal Medicine* 2017;30:2742–6. https://doi.org/10.1080/14767058.2016.1261401.

[42] Jenabi E, Fereidooni B. The uterine leiomyoma and placenta previa: a meta-analysis. *J. Matern. Fetal Neonatal. Med.* 2019; 32:1200–4. https://doi.org/10.1080/14767058.2017.14000 03.

[43] Rosati P, Exacoustòs C, Mancuso S. Longitudinal evaluation of uterine myoma growth during pregnancy. A sonographic study. *J. Ultrasound Med.* 1992;11:511–5. https://doi.org/10.7863/jum.1992.11.10.511.

[44] Winer-Muram HT, Muram D, Gillieson MS, Ivey B J, Muggah H F. Uterine myomas in pregnancy. *Can. Med. Assoc. J.* 1983;128:949–50.

[45] Aharoni A, Reiter A, Golan D, Paltiely Y, Sharf M. Patterns of growth of uterine leiomyomas during pregnancy. A prospective longitudinal study. *Br. J. Obstet. Gynaecol.* 1988;95:510–3. https://doi.org/10.1111/j.1471-0528.1988.tb12807.x.

[46] Takamoto N, Leppert P C, Yu S Y. Cell death and proliferation and its relation to collagen degradation in uterine involution of rat. *Connect. Tissue Res.* 1998;37:163–75. https://doi.org/10.3109/ 0300 8209809002436.

[47] Terry K L, De Vivo I, Hankinson S E, Missmer S A. Reproductive characteristics and risk of uterine leiomyomata. *Fertil Steril* 2010;94:2703–7. https://doi.org/10.1016/j.fertnstert.2010.04.065.

[48] Laughlin S K, Hartmann K E, Baird D D. Postpartum factors and natural fibroid regression. *Am. J. Obstet. Gynecol.* 2011;204: 496.e1-6. https://doi.org/10.1016/j.ajog.2011.02.018.

[49] Di Spiezio Sardo A, Di Carlo C, Minozzi S, Spinelli M, Pistotti V, Alviggi C, et al. Efficacy of hysteroscopy in improving reproductive outcomes of infertile couples: a systematic review and meta-analysis. *Hum. Reprod. Update* 2016;22:479–96. https:// doi.org/10.1093/humupd/dmw008.

[50] American Association of Gynecologic Laparoscopists (AAGL): Advancing Minimally Invasive Gynecology Worldwide. AAGL practice report: practice guidelines for the diagnosis and management of submucous leiomyomas. *J. Minim. Invasive Gynecol.* 2012;19:152–71. https://doi.org/10.1016/j.jmig.2011. 09.005.

[51] Purohit P, Vigneswaran K. Fibroids and Infertility. *Curr. Obstet. Gynecol. Rep.* 2016;5:81–8. https://doi.org/10.1007/s13669-016-0162-2.

[52] Metwally M, Raybould G, Cheong YC, Horne AW. Surgical treatment of fibroids for subfertility. *Cochrane Database Syst. Rev.* 2020; 1:CD003857. https://doi.org/10.1002/14651858. CD003857. pub4.

[53] Aas-Eng M K, Langebrekke A, Hudelist G. Complications in operative hysteroscopy - is prevention possible? *Acta Obstet. Gynecol. Scand.* 2017;96:1399–403. https://doi.org/10.1111/aogs. 13209.

[54] Palomba S, Zupi E, Russo T, Falbo A, Marconi D, Tolino A, et al. A multicenter randomized, controlled study comparing laparoscopic versus minilaparotomic myomectomy: short-term outcomes. *Fertil. Steril.* 2007;88:942–51. https://doi.org/10.1016/j.fertnstert.2006.12.048.

[55] Palomba S, Fornaciari E, Falbo A, La Sala G B. Safety and efficacy of the minilaparotomy for myomectomy: a systematic review and meta-analysis of randomized and non-randomized controlled trials. *Reprod. Biomed.* Online 2015;30:462–81. https://doi.org/10.1016/j.rbmo.2015.01.013.

[56] Alessandri F, Lijoi D, Mistrangelo E, Ferrero S, Ragni N. Randomized study of laparoscopic versus minilaparotomic myomectomy for uterine myomas. *J. Minim. Invasive Gynecol.* 2006;13:92–7. https://doi.org/10.1016/j.jmig.2005.11.008.

[57] Hartmann K E, Fonnesbeck C, Surawicz T, Krishnaswami S, Andrews J C, Wilson J E, et al. *Management of Uterine Fibroids.* Agency for Healthcare Research and Quality (US); 2017.

[58] Tanos V, Berry K E, Frist M, Campo R, DeWilde R L. Prevention and Management of Complications in Laparoscopic Myomectomy. *Biomed. Res. Int.* 2018;2018:8250952. https://doi.org/10.1155/2018/8250952.

[59] Kongnyuy E J, Broek N van den, Wiysonge C S. A systematic review of randomized controlled trials to reduce hemorrhage during myomectomy for uterine fibroids. *International Journal of Gynecology & Obstetrics* 2008;100:4–9. https://doi.org/10.1016/j.ijgo.2007.05.050.

[60] Fukuda M, Tanaka T, Kamada M, Hayashi A, Yamashita Y, Terai Y, et al. Comparison of the perinatal outcomes after laparoscopic myomectomy versus abdominal myomectomy. *Gynecol. Obstet. Invest.* 2013;76:203–8. https://doi.org/10.1159/000355098.

[61] Milazzo G N, Catalano A, Badia V, Mallozzi M, Caserta D. Myoma and myomectomy: Poor evidence concern in pregnancy.

J. Obstet. Gynaecol. Res. 2017;43:1789–804. https://doi.org/10.1111/jog.13437.

[62] Zhang Y, Hua K Q. Patients' age, myoma size, myoma location, and interval between myomectomy and pregnancy may influence the pregnancy rate and live birth rate after myomectomy. *J. Laparoendosc. Adv. Surg. Tech.* A 2014;24:95–9. https://doi.org/10.1089/lap.2013.0490.

[63] Tsuji S, Takahashi K, Imaoka I, Sugimura K, Miyazaki K, Noda Y. *MRI Evaluation of the Uterine Structure after Myomectomy.* GOI 2006;61:106–10. https://doi.org/10.1159/000089144.

[64] Takahashi N, Harada M, Tanabe R, Takayanagi A, Izumi G, Oi N, et al. Factors associated with successful pregnancy in women of late reproductive age with uterine fibroids who undergo embryo cryopreservation before surgery. *Journal of Obstetrics and Gynaecology Research* 2018;44:1956–62. https://doi.org/10.1111/jog.13754.

[65] Gambacorti-Passerini Z, Gimovsky A C, Locatelli A, Berghella V. Trial of labor after myomectomy and uterine rupture: a systematic review. *Acta Obstet. Gynecol. Scand.* 2016;95:724–34. https://doi.org/10.1111/aogs.12920.

[66] Gambacorti-Passerini Z M, Penati C, Carli A, Accordino F, Ferrari L, Berghella V, et al. Vaginal birth after prior myomectomy. *Eur. J. Obstet. Gynecol. Reprod. Biol.* 2018;231:198–203. https://doi.org/10.1016/j.ejogrb.2018.10.007.

[67] Liu Q-W, Han T, Yang M, Tong X-W, Wang J-J. A systematic review on efficacy and safety of gasless laparoscopy in the management of uterine leiomyoma. *J. Huazhong Univ. Sci. Technol Med. Sci.* 2016;36:142–9. https://doi.org/10.1007/s11596-016-1557-z.

[68] Iavazzo C, Mamais I, Gkegkes I D. Robotic assisted vs laparoscopic and/or open myomectomy: systematic review and meta-analysis of the clinical evidence. *Arch. Gynecol. Obstet.* 2016;294:5–17. https://doi.org/10.1007/s00404-016-4061-6.

[69] Takmaz O, Ozbasli E, Gundogan S, Bastu E, Batukan C, Dede S, et al. Symptoms and Health Quality After Laparoscopic and Robotic Myomectomy. *JSLS* 2018;22. https://doi.org/10.4293/JSLS.2018.00030.

[70] Zupi E, Centini G, Sabbioni L, Lazzeri L, Argay I M, Petraglia F. Nonsurgical Alternatives for Uterine Fibroids. *Best Pract. Res. Clin. Obstet. Gynaecol.* 2016;34:122–31. https://doi.org/10.1016/j.bpobgyn.2015.11.013.

[71] Donnez J, Arriagada P, Donnez O, Dolmans M-M. Emerging treatment options for uterine fibroids. *Expert. Opin. Emerg. Drugs* 2018;23:17–23. https://doi.org/10.1080/14728214.2018.1446943.

[72] Donnez J, Arriagada P, Donnez O, Dolmans M-M. Current management of myomas: the place of medical therapy with the advent of selective progesterone receptor modulators. *Curr. Opin. Obstet. Gynecol.* 2015;27:422–31. https://doi.org/10.1097/GCO.0000000000000229.

[73] Tsigkou A, Reis F M, Lee M H, Jiang B, Tosti C, Centini G, et al. Increased progesterone receptor expression in uterine leiomyoma: correlation with age, number of leiomyomas, and clinical symptoms. *Fertil. Steril.* 2015;104:170-175.e1. https://doi.org/10.1016/j.fertnstert.2015.04.024.

[74] Morgante G, Centini G, Troìa L, Orvieto R, De Leo V. Ulipristal acetate before in vitro fertilization: efficacy in infertile women with submucous fibroids. *Reprod. Biol. Endocrinol.* 2020;18. https://doi.org/10.1186/s12958-020-00611-1.

[75] Sancho J M, Delgado V S de la C, Valero M J N, Soteras M G, Amate V P, Carrascosa A A. Hysteroscopic myomectomy outcomes after 3-month treatment with either Ulipristal Acetate or GnRH analogues: a retrospective comparative study. *European Journal of Obstetrics and Gynecology and Reproductive Biology* 2016;198:127–30. https://doi.org/10.1016/j.ejogrb.2016.01.014.

[76] Dolmans M-M, Donnez J, Fellah L. Uterine fibroid management: Today and tomorrow. *Journal of Obstetrics and Gynaecology Research* 2019;45:1222–9. https://doi.org/10.1111/jog.14002.

[77] Donnez J, Vázquez F, Tomaszewski J, Nouri K, Bouchard P, Fauser BCJM, et al. Long-term treatment of uterine fibroids with ulipristal acetate ☆. *Fertil. Steril.* 2014;101:1565-1573.e1-18. https://doi.org/10.1016/j.fertnstert.2014.02.008.

[78] Donnez J, Donnez O, Matule D, Ahrendt H-J, Hudecek R, Zatik J, et al. Long-term medical management of uterine fibroids with ulipristal acetate. *Fertil. Steril.* 2016;105:165-173.e4. https://doi.org/10.1016/j.fertnstert.2015.09.032.

[79] Williams A R W, Bergeron C, Barlow D H, Ferenczy A. Endometrial morphology after treatment of uterine fibroids with the selective progesterone receptor modulator, ulipristal acetate. *Int. J. Gynecol. Pathol.* 2012;31:556–69. https://doi.org/10.1097/PGP.0b013e318251035b.

[80] *Suspension of ulipristal acetate for uterine fibroids during ongoing EMA review liver injury risk.* European Medicines Agency 2020. https://www.ema.europa.eu/en/news/suspension-ulipristal-acetate-uterine-fibroids-during-ongoing-ema-review-liver-injury-risk (accessed June 2, 2020).

[81] Bulun S E. Uterine fibroids. *N. Engl. J. Med.* 2013;369:1344–55. https://doi.org/10.1056/NEJMra1209993.

[82] Islam M S, Protic O, Stortoni P, Grechi G, Lamanna P, Petraglia F, et al. Complex networks of multiple factors in the pathogenesis of uterine leiomyoma. *Fertil. Steril.* 2013;100:178–93. https://doi.org/10.1016/j.fertnstert.2013.03.007.

[83] Marsh E E, Chibber S, W u J, Siegersma K, Kim J, Bulun S. Epidermal growth factor-containing fibulin-like extracellular matrix protein 1 expression and regulation in uterine leiomyoma. *Fertil. Steril.* 2016;105:1070–5. https://doi.org/10.1016/j.fertnstert.2015.12.004.

[84] Protic O, Toti P, Islam M S, Occhini R, Giannubilo S R, Catherino W H, et al. Possible involvement of inflammatory/reparative processes in the development of uterine fibroids. *Cell Tissue Res.* 2016;364:415–27. https://doi.org/10.1007/s00441-015-2324-3.

[85] Yin P, Ono M, Moravek M B, Coon J S, Navarro A, Monsivais D, et al. Human uterine leiomyoma stem/progenitor cells expressing CD34 and CD49b initiate tumors in vivo. *J. Clin. Endocrinol. Metab.* 2015;100:E601-606. https://doi.org/10.1210/jc.2014-2134.

[86] Parsanezhad M E, Azmoon M, Alborzi S, Rajaeefard A, Zarei A, Kazerooni T, et al. A randomized, controlled clinical trial comparing the effects of aromatase inhibitor (letrozole) and gonadotropin-releasing hormone agonist (triptorelin) on uterine leiomyoma volume and hormonal status. *Fertil. Steril.* 2010;93:192–8. https://doi.org/10.1016/j.fertnstert.2008.09.064.

[87] Seitz C, Bumbuliene Ž, Costa A R, Heikinheimo O, Heweker A, Hudeček R, et al. Rationale and design of ASTEROID 2, a randomized, placebo- and active comparator-controlled study to assess the efficacy and safety of vilaprisan in patients with uterine fibroids. *Contemp. Clin. Trials.* 2017;55:56–62. https://doi.org/10.1016/j.cct.2017.02.002.

In: Uterine Fibroids …   ISBN: 978-1-53619-184-4
Editors: Marco Mitidieri et al.   © 2021 Nova Science Publishers, Inc.

Chapter 3

UTERINE FIBROIDS AND PREGNANCY: LAST INSIGHTS

Alessandra Carosi, Giovanni Ruspa, MD and Marta Tosi*

SC Ostetricia e Ginecologia, Ospedale SS Trinità,
Borgomanero, Italy

ABSTRACT

Fibroids are the most common benign solid tumor of the female genital tract.

Although leiomyomas are usually asymptomatic during pregnancy however they may complicate its course.

Fibroids increase in size during early pregnancy and then decrease in the third trimester.

Determination of number, size, location and relationship to placenta implantation of myomas in the first trimester of pregnancy is very important because this may modify the related obstetric risk.

---

* Corresponding Author's E-mail: Alessandra Carosi. (alessandracarosi@alice.it).

Uterine fibroids increase the risk of cesarean delivery but the majority of patients have a successful vaginal delivery. They increase also fetal malpresentation, labor dystocia, abruption placenta and post-partum hemorrhage.

Surgical management of uterine leiomyoma during pregnancy is not usual because of its complications but may be successfully performed in carefully selected patients.

The hypothetical risk of uterine rupture during pregnancy appears similar after both myomectomy and cesarean section (CS) and is due to the presence of scar tissue.

Pregnant women with previous myomectomy could be managed similarly to those with previous CS with trial of labor.

INTRODUCTION

Fibroid, myoma, and leiomyoma are synonymous to define the most common benign solid tumor of the female genital tract, whose prevalence increases with age, peaking in women in their 40s. The exact incidence is difficult to calculate, as they may be asymptomatic and diagnosed only incidentally [1]. The prevalence is approximately 2%, ranging from 0.1% to 12.5%, and differs with ethnicity (18% in African - American women, 8% in white women, and 10% in Hispanic women) [2]. However, up to 50% that are asymptomatic may have significant social and economic impact, and may affect women's quality of life negatively.

Clinical symptoms include menstrual abnormalities, anemia, bladder dysfunction, pelvic pain, and fertility problems. Although most women with uterine fibroids have a regular pregnancy, data from the literature suggest that they are associated with a higher risk of spontaneous miscarriage, preterm labor, placental abruption, fetal malpresentation, labor dystocia, cesarean delivery, postpartum hemorrhage and hysterectomy [3, 4], Table 1 [3].

The most important factors in determining morbidity in pregnancy include fibroid number, size, location, and relationship to placenta implantation [2, 7].

Table 1. Cumulative obstetrics outcomes from included studies*

	Fibroids	No Fibroids	P	Unadjusted OR (95% CI)
Cesarean	48.8%	13.3%	< 0.001	3.7 (3.5-3.9)
Malpresentation	13.0%	4.5%	< 0.001	2.9 (2.6-3.2)
Labor dystocia	7.5%	3.1%	< 0.001	2.4 (2.1-2.7)
Postpartum hemorrhage	2.5%	1.4%	< 0.001	1.8 (1.4-2.2)
IUGR	11.2%	8.6%	< 0.001	1.4 (1.1-1.7)
Abruption	3.0%	0.9%	< 0.001	3.2 (2.6-4.0)

* While in the study of Dima Ezzadine et All [4] in the group of women with fibroids the risk of PROM was not increased compared to the control group, according to Vitale et All [5] uterine fibroids are a risk factor for PROM and PPROM . Large uterine fibroids are significantly associated with PPROM [6].

Fibroids significantly increase in size during early pregnancy and then decrease in the third trimester. The mean increase in fibroid volume during pregnancy is 12%, and very few fibroids increase by > 25%.(8) It is widely thought that myomas grow rapidly during pregnancy under the influence of hormone stimulation and increased blood flow. According to the current evidence, the rapid exponential increase in serum human chorionic gonadotropin (hCG) in the first weeks of pregnancy until 12 weeks and the particular kinetics of its receptor may explain the similar rapid growth trend of fibroids [2].

Ultrasonographic evalutation before and during pregnancy is the best tool to determination not only the size, but also the number, location and ultrasound features of myoma, its relationship with the area of placental insertion and its vascularization [1].

After precise determination of number, size and location of myomas during the first trimester, frequently ultrasound controls should be performed, because myoma growth may modify the related obstetric risk [2].

PREGNANCY

Pregnancy with myomas is at a higher risk for obstetric complications than pregnancy without myomas because myomas have been associated with an increased risk for miscarriage, pelvic pain, premature rupture of membranes, preterm delivery, placental abruption, dysfunctional birth, fetal malpresentation, dystocia, cesarean birth, intrauterine fetal demise (IUFD) and intrauterine growth restriction (IUGR).

Fibroids may have a small effect on fetal growth (OR 1.4; 95% CI, 1.1-1.7) [9]. Recent evidence indicates an increased risk of small for gestational age (SGA) with retroplacental leiomyomas > 4 cm that can interfere with placentation [2].

Indirectly, fibroid location and size may further increase the rate of cesarean birth, affecting uterine vascular and contractile activity. Large myomas (mostly defined as > 5cm) are associated with an increased risk of pPROM, premature delivery and blood loss at delivery; large uterine leiomyomas (approx. 10 cm) may induce restriction of the uterine cavity, causing fetal deformities from long-term compressive force [2].

The anatomic anomalies described in the literature are limb reduction, caudal dysplasia, head deformation and congenital torticollis [10].

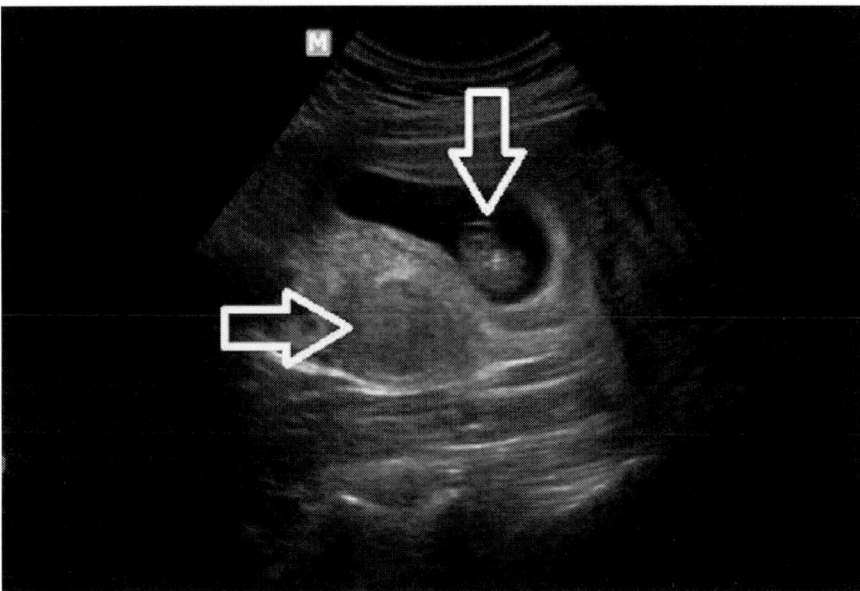

Figure 1. An early intrauterine pregnancy (gestational sac and embryo-vertical arrow) located in a uterus with an intramural fibroid (horizontal arrow).

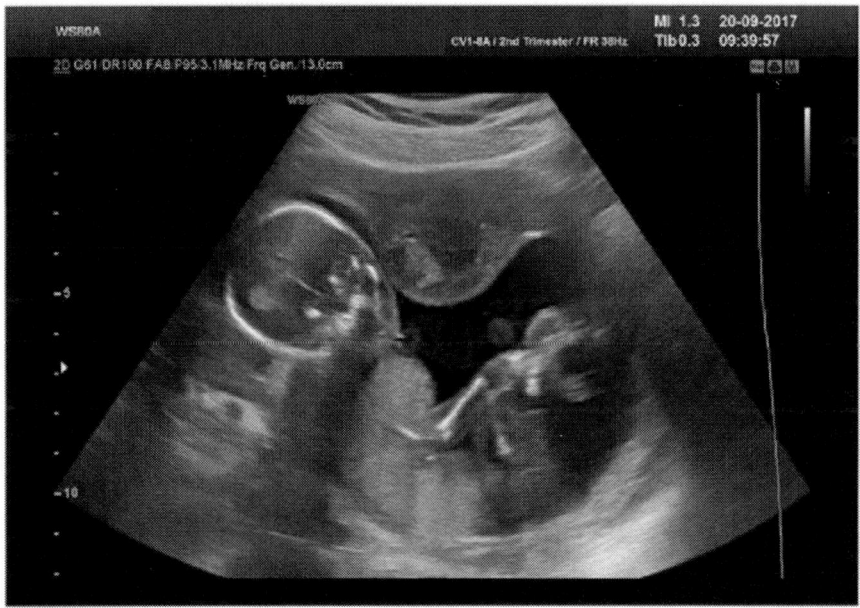

Figure 2. Viable fetus in the uterine cavity 24 th week of the pregnancy. Uterine fibroid located in the anterior wall.

LABOUR AND POST-PARTUM

Studies have consistently reported that uterine fibroids are associated with an increased risk of cesarean delivery (OR 3.7; 95%IC,3.5-3.9) [9] especially when the fibroids are located in the lower uterine segment [4, 11]. Although the presence of a large myoma is not an indication for Cesarean Section before labor, in clinical practice it has possibly lowered the threshold to proceed with the abdominal route of delivery when other obstetric complications are present. Large fibroids or multiple fibroids are not an immediate contraindication to labor if women are eligible for vaginal delivery [2].

There is a lack of knowledge and basic research on the effect of fibroid on labor however fibroids may physically impede the propagation of contraction waves throughout the uterus; furthermore they lack prostaglandin receptors, essential for physiological uterine peristalsis. The uterus with fibroid(s), however, is no less responsive to the use of oxytocics [2, 12]. The majority of patients have a successful vaginal delivery, except in the case of cervical or anterior isthmic fibroid. Large and multiple fibroids distorting the uterine cavity have been consistently associated with fetal malpresentation and large previa myomas may block the passage required for vaginal delivery. Nowadays ultrasound is fundamental for establishing the modality of delivery before labor onset: the vaginal delivery cannot be carried out if myoma is located between the fetal head and the internal os, interfering with both cervical dilatation and fetal head descent. [2, 12].

The risk of post-partum hemorrhage (PPH) is twofold higher than in the general population [2, 7]. Decreased uterine contractility and uncoordinated contractions may lead to inefficient myometrial retraction in the third stage of labor. The increasing size and the location of fibroids in the lower part increase the risk of PPH. Retroplacental submucous myomas increase not only the risk of PPH but also that of retained and adherent placenta. Rarely myomas may obstruct the passage of lochia and induce uterine atony for hematometra. It is advisable to organize a care plan for PPH prophylaxis in women with fibroids [2, 12].

In guideline: "Emorragia del postpartum come prevenirla, come curarla," Obstetric Surveillance System (ItOSS) 2016, in "Prevention and Management of Postpartum Haemorrahge," Green-top Guideline No. 52, December 2016, BJOG – RCOG and "Intrapartum care for healthy women and babies Clinical guideline," December 2014 Last updated: February 2017, fibroids are not considered risk factor for PPH.

CESAREAN SECTION

In C-section the usual practice is to keep away from the fibroid and choose the best accessible incision line at least 2 cm from the fibroid margin. If possible, a lower segment CS is preferred. In cases of myoma involving the lower segment many surgeons prefer the classic CS instead of low transverse CS, others prefer to perform a myomectomy at the time of CS, before fetus delivery.

The operation is technically challenging with difficult intraoperative hemostasis and is associated with a higher incidence of postoperative complications.

The risk of PPH is higher in cesarean delivery [2, 12].

MYOMECTOMY IN PREGNANCY

Surgeons usually hesitate to perform myomectomy in pregnancy because of the increased uterine blood flow and volume during gestation, which raise the risk of hemorrhagic complications and increase the likelihood of hysterectomy, while the uterine manipulation can predispose toward adverse pregnancy outcomes [2]. However, myomectomy in pregnancy can be considered as an option for selected cases. Urgent myomectomy is related mainly to a torsion of a pedunculated myoma or to rare cases of necrosis and consequent inflammatory peritoneal reaction [1, 16].

Other indications for myomectomy in pregnancy are recurrent or severe pain, which have failed to be treated by conservative management after the first trimester, rapid growth of myoma, large fibroids located in the lower uterine segment or if they deform the placentation site, and large fibroid causing compression phenomena with intestinal obstruction or subobstruction. Absolute contraindications to myomectomy are uterine atony, intramural nodules growing and expanding toward the uterine cavity, or displacing large vessels.

There is evidence that myomectomy could be performed during every trimester. Most of the studies in the literature report a preference of the laparoscopic approach for the treatment of fibroids in pregnancy [17] and myomectomy during cesarean section is still controversial, even though a well tolerated and feasible procedure [1, 17].

Routine myomectomy should be abandoned, but it could be considered only in selected patients with careful consideration of different factors: uterine contraction, size, number, and location of myomas in comparison with large vessels and presence of placenta accreta/increta. Routine myomectomy has to be executed only if unavoidable to facilitate safe delivery of the fetus or closure of the uterine breach.

Cesarean miomectomy is generally considered relatively safe in cases of anterior wall myomas, subserous and pedunculated myomas, particularly if a myomectomy is feasible without additional hysterotomy [18]. Particularly, the experience of the surgeon and the presence of a tertiary center have to be considered, because a correct myomectomy during cesarean birth requires special technical care about incision orientation, recognition and preparation of cleavage plain, hemostasis, and sutures [1, 19]. Multiple myomas, deep intramural, fundal and cornual myomas and posterior uterine wall myomas are associated with more surgical complications during cesarean miomectomy [18].

Comparable studies have combined myomectomy during cesarean delivery with the use of preventive measures for hemorrhage. These measures included pre-operative embolization of uterine arteries, intraoperativeuse of a tourniquet, or uterine artery devascularization. However, the most common practice was to administer high doses of oxytocin intra and postoperatively, and most studies have not required any techniques beyond the use of oxytocin. Furthermore, oxytocin and the additionaldoses of uterotonics (oxytocin and/or prostaglandins) were used in accordance with international guidelines intra and postoperatively, in case of uterine atony, which was regarded as an adverse outcome itself [20].

PREGNANCY WITH A PRIOR MYOMECTOMY OR C-SECTION

Uterine rupture during labor in patients with a prior myomectomy has been reported; however, the magnitude of this risk and the specific risk factors associated with it are difficult to ascertain [4].

The hypothetical risk of uterine rupture during pregnancy is due to the presence of scar tissue; therefore any previous surgical interventions on the uterus are considered a risk factor for uterine ropture. This risk appears similar after both myomectomy and C-section [2]. Most cases of uterine rupture occur in the third trimester or during labor, when intrauterine pressure is more elevated.

The repair process after myomectomy is fundamental to preserve uterine integrity and depends on the general status of the patient, enucleation technique, use of electrocoagulation, formation of hematoma and type of suture. The establishment of an adequate interval period is problematic: some studies suggested a period between 2 and

12 weeks, others, 12 months; while others concluded that there is no safe interval.

A previous C-Section or any other conditions of myometrial damage represent a risk of placenta accreta [2]. Although the risk appears to be low, an ultrasound examination is recommended in the late second or early third trimester to look for evidence of abnormal placentation [4].

The presence of uterine scars creates an area of substitution of the muscle tissue with a fibroid tissue that causes reduced capacity for contraction during and after delivery, and indeed, significant blood loss at delivery in pregnant women with previous myomectomy has been reported.

Most women with a previous myomectomy were more likely to require C-Section to minimize the risk of uterine-rupture.

According to the literature, however, CS is advisable when > 50% of the myometrium is involved during myomectomy when a multiple myomectomy is performed and when myomectomy has created a large defect in the active segment of the uterus. Careful management of labor is a prerequisite to ensure low risk of maternal complications and good perinatal outcome. Pregnant women with previous myomectomy could be managed similarly to those with previous CS with trial of labor [2].

CONCLUSION

Uterine fibroids are common in reproductive age women. Most women with fibroids will have an uneventful pregnancy. However, multiple fibroids, large size (> 3 cm), and submucosal and retroplacental location are risk factors for adverse pregnancy events, including miscarriage, placental abruption, and preterm labor and birth. Myomectomy should be avoided during pregnancy because of the risk of significant morbidity. Most women with fibroids will have a successful vaginal delivery and should therefore be offered a trial of labor. Cesarean delivery should be reserved for standard obstetrical indications [4].

REFERENCES

[1] Management of uterine fibroids in pregnancy: recent trends. Vitale SG, Padula F, Gulino FA. *Curr. Opin. Obstet. Gynecol.* 2015 Dec; 27 PMID: 26485457 Review.

[2] Myoma and myomectomy: Poor evidence concern in pregnancy. Milazzo GN, Catalano A, Badia V, Mallozzi M, Caserta D. *J. Obstet. Gynaecol. Res.* 2017 Dec;43(12):1789-1804. doi: 10.1111/jog.13437. Epub 2017 Sep 11. PMID: 28892210 Review.

[3] Contemporary Management of Fibroids in Pregnancy Hee Joong Lee, MD, PhD,1 Errol R Norwitz, MD, PhD, 2 and Julia Shaw, MD, *MBA Rev. Obstet. Gynecol.* 2010.

[4] Are Women With Uterine Fibroids at Increased Risk for Adverse Pregnancy Outcome? Ezzedine D., and Norwitz E.R. *Clinical obstetrics and gynecology*, marzo 2016.

[5] Management of uterine leiomyomas in pregnancy: review of literature. Salvatore Giovanni Vitale, Alessandro Tropea, Diego Rossetti, Marco Carnelli e Antonio Cianci, *Updates in Surgery* 2013.

[6] Neonatal outcomes in women with sonographically identified uterine leiomyomata. Lai J, Caughey AB, Qidwai GI, Jacoby AF. *J. Matern. Fetal Neonatal. Med.* 2012.

[7] Pregnancy outcome and uterine fibroids. Parazzini F, Tozzi L, Bianchi S. Best Pract Res Clin Obstet Gynaecol. 2016 Jul; *Epub* 2015 Nov 25. PMID: 26723475 Review.

[8] The impact of uterine leyomyomas on reproductive outcomes. Cook H, Ezzati M, Segars JH, McCarthy K. *Minerva Ginecol.* 2010.

[9] Fibroids and reproductive outcomes: a systematic literature review from conception to delivery. Klatsky PC, Tran ND, Caughey AB, Fujimoto VY. *Am. J. Obstet. Gynecol.* 2008.

[10] Increased risk of preterm births among women with uterine leiomyoma: a nationwide population-based study. Chen YH, Lin HC, Chen SF, Lin HC. *Hum Reprod.* 2009 Dec.

[11] Large uterine leiomyomata and risk of cesarean delivery. Vergani P, Locatelli A, Ghidini A, Andreani M, Sala F, Pezzullo JC. *Obstet. Gynecol.* 2007.

[12] Vaginal Myomectomy for Semipedunculated Cervical Myoma During Pregnancy Mikitaka Obara, Yuko Hatakeyama, Yasushi Shimizu. *AJP Rep.*, Epub 2014.

[13] Emorragia del postpartum come prevenirla, come curarla, *Obstetric Surveillance System* (ItOSS) 2016.

[14] Prevention and Management of Postpartum Haemorrahge," Green-top Guideline No. 52, December 2016, *BJOG – RCOG.*

[15] Intrapartum care for healthy women and babies Clinical guideline," December 2014 Last updated: February 2017, *fibroids are not considered risk factor for PPH.*

[16] Laparoscopic Approach to Fibroid Torsion Presenting as an Acute Abdomen in Pregnancy Andrew Currie, Elizabeth Bradley, Marcus McEwen, Nawar Al-Shabibi, Peter D Willson. *JSLS* 2013.

[17] *Prise en charge des myomes utérins durant la grossesse. Revue de la littérature Management of uterine myomas during pregnancy* F. Levast, G.Legendre, P.-E. Bouet, L. Sentilhes 2016.

[18] Cesarean myomectomy trends and controversies: an appraisal Radmila Sparić, Antonio Malvasi, Saša Kadija, Ivana Babović, Lazar Nejković, Andrea Tinelli. *The Journal of Maternal-Fetal & Neonatal Medicine* 2017.

[19] Cesarean myomectomy in modern obstetrics: More light and fewer shadows Radmila Sparić, Saša Kadija, Aleksandar Stefanović, Svetlana Spremović Radjenović, Ivana Likić Ladjević, Jela Popović, Andrea Tinelli. *Obstetrcs and Ginaecology* 2017.

[20] Outcome and risk factors of cesarean deliverywith and without cesarean myomectomy in women with uterinemyomatasI. Dedes. L. Scha'ffer, R. Zimmermann, T. Burkhardt, C. Haslinge. *Arch. Gynecol. Obstet.* 2017.

In: Uterine Fibroids ...
Editors: Marco Mitidieri et al.

ISBN: 978-1-53619-184-4
© 2021 Nova Science Publishers, Inc.

Chapter 4

MEDICAL TREATMENT OF UTERINE FIBROIDS

Maria Grazia Baù[1], MD and Alessandra Surace[2,], MD*
[1]SCDO Ginecologia ed ostetricia 3, Sant'Anna Hospital,
Città della salute e della Scienza, Turin, Italy
[2]SCDU Ginecologia ed ostetricia 2, Sant'Anna Hospital,
Città della salute e della Scienza, Turin, Italy

ABSTRACT

Medical therapy can be used as an alternative to surgery or as a pre-operative ancillary. Various medical options are currently available to manage symptomatic uterine UFs. The choice of the appropriate therapeutic approach for UFs depends on several factors, including women's age, childbearing aspirations, extent and severity of symptoms, size, number and location of myomas, risk of malignancy and proximity to menopause. Nonsteroidal Anti-Inflammatory Drugs (NSAIDs), tranexamic acid, Gonadotropin-Releasing Hormone (GnRH) agonists (leuprolide acetate, goserelin acetate and nafarelin acetate),

---

[*] Corresponding Author's E-mail: alessandra.sur@gmail.com.

Gonadotropin-Releasing Hormone (GnRH) antagonists (cetrorelix acetate and ganirelix acetate), Selective Progesterone Receptor Modulators (SPRMs), oral progestogens, levonorgestrel intrauterine device, danazol, Aromatase inhibitors and Raloxifene are the current therapeutic options for UFs management. Also natural compounds could improve symptoms management of UFs. Medical treatments are confirmed to be safe and effective in reducing the symptoms and the size of the UFs, avoiding or postponing surgery and preserving fertility. And the benefits are not limited to patients: as cost-effectiveness studies confirm, medical treatment proves to be the most advantageous therapeutic option also from a pharmacoeconomic point of view, with savings for the national health system estimated at around 45 million euro per year.

INTRODUCTION

Pharmacological therapy can be used as an alternative to surgery or as a pre-operative ancillary to improve and optimize surgical outcomes by reducing size of uterine fibroids (UFs) and/or uterine bleeding. It may be used as 'stand-alone' treatment for temporary short-term relief of symptoms, such as in the case of women with symptomatic UFs in the pre-menopausal years or in patients not suitable for surgery due to medical reasons. Several therapeutic options are available for treating these patients that are confirmed to be safe and effective in reducing the symptoms and the size of the UFs. And the benefits are not limited to patients: as cost-effectiveness studies confirm, medical treatment proves to be the most advantageous therapeutic option also from a pharmacoeconomic point of view, with savings for the national health system estimated at around 45 million euro per year.

NONSTEROIDAL ANTI-INFLAMMATORY DRUGS (NSAIDS)

NSAIDs cause the inhibition of the enzyme cyclooxygenase, which diminishes the production of prostaglandins. A Cochrane review evaluating the effectiveness of NSAIDs in the management of abnormal uterine bleeding/heavy menstrual bleeding included 18 studies [1]. The authors found the use of NSAIDs was superior to placebo but less effective than tranexamic acid, danazol or the levonorgestrel releasing intrauterine device when evaluating the therapeutic impact on abnormal uterine bleeding. Despite their usefulness with reducing both dysmenorrhea and blood loss, these agents have not been shown to lead to dissolution of the UFs, being considered as only symptomatic relievers. In the case of women suffering from abnormal uterine bleeding or heavy menstrual bleeding, medical management NSAIDs, progestin, combination of oral contraceptives, a levonorgestrel releasing intrauterine device, or tranexamic acid has been shown to be beneficial [2].

TRANEXAMIC ACID

The antifibrinolytic tranexamic acid at a dose of 1 g every 6 hours reduces bleeding by 9% in uterine leiomyomas and up to 95% with menorrhagia alone [3].

GONADOTROPIN-RELEASING HORMONE (GNRH) AGONISTS (LEUPROLIDE ACETATE, GOSERELIN ACETATE AND NAFARELIN ACETATE)

As a class of medication, GnRH agonists have historically been considered the most effective presurgical therapy for symptomatic UFs. They induce a "menopausal" hypoestrogenic status (by downregulation of the hypothalamic-pituitary-ovarian axis), amenorrhea, improvement in symptoms and rapid reduction in leiomyoma volume. The benefits are counterbalanced with unavoidable side effect profile: vasomotor symptoms, vaginal dryness, sleep disturbances, myalgia, arthralgia, mood-swings, and potential cognitive impairment [4, 5]. Long-term therapy, greater than 6 months, with GnRH agonists has been implicated in bone loss of approximately 6% [6]. Important to note, both the benefits and side effects of GnRH agonists are temporary and reverse with the discontinuation of the medication [7]. In one of the large scale clinical trials assessing leuprolide efficacy in women with symptomatic UFs, 128 women were enrolled and placed into either the treatment or placebo arm. Those in the treatment arm received 3.75 mg leuprolide acetate intramuscularly monthly for a total of 6 months. The authors found a 36% reduction in uterine volume at 12 weeks and 45% with 24 weeks of treatment. However, mean uterine volume returned to pretreatment size 24 week after cessation of leuprolide acetate [8]. However, given the hypoestrogenic state and bone loss, most organizations including the American Congress of Obstetricians and Gynecologist (ACOG) recommend limiting the use of leuprolide acetate to symptomatic women scheduled to undergo surgery within 6 months of initiating therapy [9]. If used longer, ACOG recommends that low dose steroidal add-back therapy be considered to minimize continued bone loss and vasomotor symptoms.

GONADOTROPIN-RELEASING HORMONE (GNRH) ANTAGONISTS (CETRORELIX ACETATE AND GANIRELIX ACETATE)

GnRH antagonists have been shown in clinical trials to reduce UFs volume, inducing a hypoestrogenic state [10]. However, these medications are injected and must be taken every 1 to 4 days because there are currently no long-acting depot forms available in the United States, which limits their usefulness with regard to the medical treatment of UFs. Others similar compounds are under research attention: Elagolix and very recently the new drug Relugolix associated with add- back therapy, with apparently good outcomes in terms of size reduction of UFs and symptoms control but a worse cost- benefits profile (more than 80.000.000 euro/years estimated). Both of them are in tablet form.

SELECTIVE PROGESTERONE RECEPTOR MODULATORS (SPRMs)

Unlike GnRH analogues, SPRMs do not have the disadvantage of inducing estrogen deficiency. Several studies have established the potential role of SPRMs in the treatment of UFs and their association with a reduction in pain, bleeding, size of UFs and overall improvement in quality of life. Ulipristal acetate (UPA), the most recent drug of this class, is an effective and well-tolerated option for the preoperative and long-term treatment of moderate and severe symptoms of UFs in women of reproductive age [11]. The PEARL I and PEARL II trials [12] have shown the ability of ulipristal acetate not only to control myoma-associated bleeding, but also to significantly decrease myoma size. A recent safety review is ongoing about liver toxicity of UPA, so EMA's safety committee has recommended women to stop taking 5-mg ulipristal acetate for uterine UFs.

STEROIDAL CONTRACEPTIVE THERAPIES (ORAL CONTRACEPTIVE, PATCHES AND RINGS)

In observational studies, these have been shown to reduce undifferentiated bleeding by 35% to 69% if used cyclically and by 87% if used continuously. They, however, do not reduce UFs size and are contraindicated in smokers aged older than 35 years.

ORAL PROGESTOGENS

They reduce UFs symptoms by 25-50%, when administered during the second part of the cycle or as 21-day contraceptives; there are no data regarding continuous administration.

LEVONORGESTREL IUD

The levonorgestrel IUD (20 mg/d) decreases the amount of UFs bleeding by up to 80% to 90% at 1 year and is an effective and safe treatment. However, its effect on the size of uterine myoma is still unclear. There is a higher expulsion rate with submucosal leiomyomas [13].

DANAZOL

Danazol induces endometrial hypotrophy and enhances UFs shrinkage, but also shows significantly more adverse effects (including weight gain, acne, musculoskeletal pain, hot flushes and hirsutism) than other medical therapies due to its androgenic action.

AROMATASE INHIBITORS

Aromatase inhibitors have been shown to readily reduce UFs size (up to 71% in 2 months) and appear to be as effective as GnRH agonist with fewer side effects; but robust evidence regarding their efficacy is lacking.

RALOXIFENE

The selective estrogen receptor modulator (SERM) raloxifene has also been investigated for treatment of symptomatic UFs; however, the few studies that are available are of low quality and provide inconsistent results.

NATURAL COMPOUNDS

More recently, the role of vitamin D, berberine, curcumin and green tee extract (epigallocatechin gallate, EGCG) was explored as potential preventive and anti-uterine fibroid options, respectively, with promising results [14].

CONCLUSION

Despite the availability of such not invasive therapies, current literature has not shown a definitive reduction in the numbers of hysterectomies performed in the United States given that most medical therapies result in a rapid return of symptoms and/or tumor volume with cessation of treatment; more over drugs available might be stratified according to price: less expensive, intermediate expensive and high expensive and the concept of cost-benefit and incremental-benefit in comparison with old drugs towards new ones, have also to be accurately taken into account.

Table 1. Comparison of recommended therapies for uterine fibroids [15]

Treatment	Description	Advantages	Disadvantages	Fertility preserved?
Medical therapies				
Gonadotropin-releasing hormone agonists[12]	Preoperative treatment to decrease size of tumors before surgery or in women approaching menopause	Decrease blood loss, operative time, and recovery time	Long-term treatment associated with higher cost, menopausal symptoms, and bone loss; increased recurrence risk with myomectomy	Depends on subsequent procedure
Levonorgestrel-releasing intrauterine system (Mirena)[13]	Treats abnormal uterine bleeding, likely by stabilization of endometrium	Most effective medical treatment for reducing blood loss; decreases fibroid volume	Irregular uterine bleeding, increased risk of device expulsion	Yes, if discontinued after resolution of symptoms
Nonsteroidal anti-inflammatory drugs[14]	Anti-inflammatories and prostaglandin inhibitors	Reduce pain and blood loss from fibroids	Do not decrease fibroid volume; gastrointestinal adverse effects	Yes
Oral contraceptives[15]	Treat abnormal uterine bleeding, likely by stabilization of endometrium	Reduce blood loss from fibroids; ease of conversion to alternate therapy if not successful	Do not decrease fibroid volume	Yes, if discontinued after resolution of symptoms
Selective progesterone receptor modulators[35,36]	Preoperative treatment to decrease size of tumors before surgery or in women approaching menopause	Decrease blood loss, operative time, and recovery time; not associated with hypoestrogenic adverse effects	Headache and breast tenderness, progesterone receptor modulator–associated endometrial changes; increased recurrence risk with myomectomy	Depends on subsequent procedure
Tranexamic acid (Cyklokapron)[37,38]	Antifibrinolytic therapy	Reduces blood loss from fibroids; ease of conversion to alternate therapy	Does not decrease fibroid volume; medical contraindications	Yes

REFERENCES

[1] Lethaby A., Duckitt K., Farquhar C. Non-steroidal anti-inflammatory drugs for heavy menstrual bleeding. *Cochrane Database of Systematic Reviews* (Online), vol. 1, p. CD000400, 2013.

[2] Practice bulletin no.136: management of abnormal uterine bleeding associated with ovulatory dysfunction. *Obstetrics & Gynecology*, vol. 122, no. 1, pp. 176-185, 2013.

[3] The North American Menopause Society (NAMS). NAMS 2018 Utian Translational Science Symposium, October 2018, San Diego, California. New therapies for leiomyomas: when surgery may not be the best option. *Menopause.* 2019; 26(9): 947-957.

[4] ACOG practice bulletin. Alternatives to hysterectomy in the management of leiomyomas. *Obstet Gynecol*, vol. 112, no. 2, Part 1, pp. 387-400, 2008.

[5] ACOG practice bulletin. *Surgical Alternatives to Hysterectomy in The Management of Leiomyomas.* Number 16, May 2000, vol.73, no. 3, pp. 285-293, 2001.

[6] Surreyand E. S. Hornstein. Prolonged GnRH agonist and add-back therapy for symptomatic endometriosis: long-term follow-up. *Obstetrics & Gynecology*, vol. 99, no. 5, pp. 709-719, 2002.

[7] Olive D. L., Lindheim S. R., Pritts E. A. Nonsurgical management of leiomyoma: impact on fertility. *Current opinion in obstetrics and gynecology*, vol. 16, no. 3, pp. 239-243, 2004.

[8] Friedman A. J., Hoffman D. I., Comite F., Browneller R. W., Miller J. D. Treatment of leiomyomata uteri with leuprolide acetate depot: a double-blind, placebo-controlled, multicenter study. The Leuprolide Study Group. *Obstet Gynecol,* vol. 77, no. 5, pp. 720-725, 1991.

[9] ACOG practice bulletin. Alternatives to hysterectomy in the management of leiomyomas. *Obstet Gynecol,* vol. 112, no. 2, Part 1, pp. 387-400, 2008.

[10] Kettel L. M., Murphy A. A., Morales A. J., Rivier J., Vale W., Yen S. S. C. Rapid regression of uterine leiomyomas in response to daily administration of gonadotropin-releasing hormone antagonist. *Fertility and Sterility,* vol. 60, no. 4, pp. 642-646, 1993.

[11] Donnez J., Arriagada P., Donnez O., Dolmans M. M. Emerging treatment options for uterine fibroids. *Expert Opin Emerg Drugs.* 2018 Mar; 23(1):17-23. doi: https://10.1080/14728214.2018. 1446943. Epub 2018 Mar 12.

[12] Faustino F., Martinho M., Reis J., Águas F. Update on medical treatment of uterine fibroids. *Eur J Obstet Gynecol Reprod Biol.* 2017 Sep; 216:61-68. doi: https://10.1016/j.ejogrb.2017.06.047. Epub 2017 Jul 8.

[13] Sayed G. H., Zakherah M. S., El-Nashar S. A., Shaaban M. M. A randomized clinical trial of a levonorgestrel-releasing intrauterine system and a low dose combined oral contraceptive for fibroid-related menorrhagia. *Int J Gynaecol Obstet* 2011; 112:126-130.

[14] Natural Compounds in the Medical Treatment of Uterine Fibroids. *J Clin Med.* 2020 May 14; 9(5). pii: E1479. doi: https://10.3390/ jcm9051479.

[15] De La Cruz M. S. D., Buchanan E. M. Uterine Fibroids: Diagnosis and Treatment. *Am Fam Physician.* 2017 Jan 15; 95(2):100-107.

In: Uterine Fibroids ... ISBN: 978-1-53619-184-4
Editors: Marco Mitidieri et al. © 2021 Nova Science Publishers, Inc.

Chapter 5

SURGICAL TREATMENT FOR UTERINE FIBROIDS

Livio Leo[1], MD, Stephanie Challancin[1], MD,
Raphael Thomasset[1], MD and Nicole Brunod[2,*], MD

[1]Obstetrics and Gynecology Department,
Beauregard Hospital, Aosta, Italy
[2]Obstetrics and Gynecology 1U, Sant'Anna Hospital,
University of Torino, Torino, Italy

ABSTRACT

Medical therapy can be used as an alternative to surgery or as a pre-operative ancillary. Various medical options are currently available to manage symptomatic uterine UFs. The choice of the appropriate therapeutic approach for UFs depends on several factors, including women's age, childbearing aspirations, extent and severity of symptoms, size, number and location of myomas, risk of malignancy and proximity to menopause. Nonsteroidal Anti-Inflammatory Drugs (NSAIDs), tranexamic acid, Gonadotropin-Releasing Hormone (GnRH) agonists

---

* Corresponding Author's E-mail: nicole.brunod@edu.unito.it.

(leuprolide acetate, goserelin acetate and nafarelin acetate), Gonadotropin-Releasing Hormone (GnRH) antagonists (cetrorelix acetate and ganirelix acetate), Selective Progesterone Receptor Modulators (SPRMs), oral progestogens, levonorgestrel intrauterine device, danazol, Aromatase inhibitors and Raloxifene are the current therapeutic options for UFs management. Also natural compounds could improve symptoms management of UFs. Medical treatments are confirmed to be safe and effective in reducing the symptoms and the size of the UFs, avoiding or postponing surgery and preserving fertility. And the benefits are not limited to patients: as cost-effectiveness studies confirm, medical treatment proves to be the most advantageous therapeutic option also from a pharmacoeconomic point of view, with savings for the national health system estimated at around 45 million euro per year.

INTRODUCTION

After a comprehensive counseling with the patient, the choice of the surgical approach depends on the volume, number and location of the fibroids. It is therefore necessary to perform an accurate mapping of all myomas using a transvaginal ultrasound possibly associated with transabdominal probe.

In women with submucosal myomas (FIGO 0-1-2) candidates for resectoscopic treatment, preoperative hysteroscopic evaluation allows the identification of the correct surgical strategy (although hysterosonography alone is often sufficient in these cases). Main elements are age, medical history and the desire for offspring.

Infertility

The key factor regarding the risk of infertility is the location of a fibroid, not its size, is the key factor regarding the risk of infertility [1]. Leiomyomas that distort the uterine cavity (submucosal or intramural with an intracavitary component) cause difficulties in conceiving and an increased risk of miscarriage [1, 2].

In contrast, a systematic review of predominantly observational studies found that infertility is not associated with the presence of subserosal fibroids and that the role of intramural fibroids is controversial [1, 2]. Since open abdominal myomectomy is performed primarily to remove intramural or subserosal myomas, its role in women with infertility is uncertain.

Leiomyomas can make it difficult or impossible to evaluate the ovaries with a pelvic exam or pelvic ultrasound. However, incorrect clinical ultrasound evaluation due to leiomyomas is not an indication for myomectomy [3]. For women in whom a uterine leiomyomatosis makes evaluation of the ovaries difficult, pelvic imaging should only be done if develop suspicious symptoms for adnexal disease (e.g., lower quadrant pelvic pain) or for women with risk factors who need to be screened for ovarian cancer. If ultrasound visualization of the ovaries is hampered by the presence of myomas, MRI should be done.

Likewise, the need to rule out the diagnosis of uterine sarcoma is not an indication for myomectomy. Uterine sarcoma is rare, and the likelihood of finding a sarcoma in women with a preoperative diagnosis of leiomyoma is much lower than the risk of serious complications associated with surgery for benign disease. In cases where sarcoma is suspected, it is necessary to complete the diagnostic process with MRI and LDH dosage.

Surgical treatment can be conservative (myomectomy) or demolitive (hysterectomy) and can be performed by laparoscopy, laparotomy or hysteroscopy. Furthermore, in selected cases, the surgery can be performed vaginally or using robotic surgery.

MYOMECTOMY AND ALTERNATIVE TREATMENTS

The choice of treatment for women with uterine leiomyomas is guided by the symptoms.

Abnormal Uterine Bleeding

Abnormal uterine bleeding in women with leiomyomas is initially treated with medical therapy (e.g., estrogen-progestogen contraceptives, tranexamic acid). If medical therapy is not sufficiently effective or tolerated, the therapeutic options include both interventional radiology procedures (uterine artery embolization, guided focused ultrasound with magnetic resonance), endometrial ablation, myomectomy and hysterectomy. The decision depends on the patient's characteristics and preferences.

Mass Related Symptoms

Treatment options for symptoms related to the mass (pain or pelvic pressure) include hysterectomy, myomectomy or interventional radiology procedures (uterine artery embolization or MRI-guided focused ultrasound). Some drug treatments (e.g., gonadotropin-releasing hormone agonists) reduce the size of the uterus but they are generally not used because chronic treatment is required, resulting in menopausal symptoms and a reduction in bone mineral density.

The choice of treatment for mass-related symptoms depends on the patient's desire to preserve fertility and/or uterine preservation and her preferences regarding definitive treatment and treatment invasiveness. The size, location of the myomas and the availability to use minimally invasive procedures are also factors that influence the decision.

Women Who Desire Pregnancy

Myomectomy is the first choice for women wishing to preserve fertility. Women who are planning a future pregnancy should be informed about obstetric problems resulting from a myomectomy. Interventional radiology procedures may not be appropriate for women planning a future pregnancy due to potential safety concerns and detrimental effects on ovarian function. For example, uterine artery embolization can adversely affect fertility and obstetric outcomes, and pregnancy safety following MRI-guided focused ultrasound therapy has not been established.

PRE-OPERATIVE PREPARING

Preparation for Any Significant Blood Loss

Myomectomy does not usually cause significant blood loss, but large fibroids or multiple formations can cause major bleeding. For patients with an increased risk of bleeding, preoperative measures such as correcting anemia or donating autologous blood can reduce the likelihood of having a blood transfusion.

Reduction in Size of Fibroids with GnRH Agonists

Preoperative use of gonadotropin-releasing hormone (GnRH) agonists offers some short-term benefits for women undergoing myomectomy with regards to blood loss and uterus size, but may increase the difficulty of surgery [9].

Myomectomy can usually be performed using a Pfannenstiel incision or, if more access is required, a Maylard incision. Compared to a large vertical incision (e.g., navel-pubic), these incisions reduce postoperative pain and improve healing [10]. In the case of large uterine size the myomectomy can be performed more easily making a transverse incision slightly higher than usual, extending the incision to the lateral edges of the rectus muscles and curving it cephalically to avoid the ileoinguinal nerves. In women with large fibroids, a vertical incision may be necessary; however, the use of GnRH agonists may reduce uterine size and allow the use of a smaller vertical or transverse incision.

A meta-analysis of 11 randomized trials showed that pre-treatment with a GnRH agonist versus placebo or no treatment before open abdominal myomectomy significantly reduced uterine size (reduction in uterine volume by 159ml) [9].

The only study that evaluated the choice of the incision found that the use of the GnRH agonist was associated with fewer vertical incisions (0 out of 13 versus 5 out of 15) [11].

The disadvantages of preoperative GnRH agonist therapy, however, outweigh the advantages for most women. Randomized studies have found that the use of these agents does not reduce the risk of blood transfusions. In addition, some surgeons have reported that the use of these drugs makes it more difficult to enuclear fibroids.

Most women undergone an abdominal myomectomy can be operated on through a Pfannenstiel incision, even for very large fibroids.

By separating the fascia from the rectus muscles, both midline and laterally, they can be further extended to give the surgeon more space to release the uterus. The use of GnRh analogs may be a reasonable option in women for whom the treatment would allow for a transverse incision instead of a longitudinal incision.

Antibiotic Prophylaxis

Myomectomy is classified as a clean procedure, as it does not involve a vaginal or intestinal incision. The American College of Obstetricians and Gynecologists (ACOG) states that antibiotic prophylaxis is not required for this procedure [12]. Other experts disagree, based on the rational that the risk of surgical site infection is likely similar to hysterectomy, for which antibiotic prophylaxis is universally recommended [13].

There are no high-quality data regarding the use of antibiotic prophylaxis in women undergoing myomectomy.

Thromboprophylaxis

Patients undergoing laparotomic myomectomy (major surgery, defined as duration > 30 minutes) have a moderate risk of venous thromboembolism and require adequate mechanical and pharmacological thromboprophylaxis. Venous compression devices are used during surgery for two to three days after surgery for all patients. Patients with an above average risk can be treated with low molecular weight heparin.

Anesthesia

Normally, laparotomic myomectomy is performed under general anesthesia, but regional spinal anesthesia can be used as well.

CONSERVATIVE SURGICAL TREATMENT: MYOMECTOMY

Since in industrialized societies the first pregnancy is more and more postponed, the finding of myomas in women of advanced reproductive age but still eager for offspring is now a frequent occurrence and, probably, is destined to be even more so in the future. The goal of conservative surgery is the removal of myomas while maintaining unchanged, sometimes improving, reproductive capacity. To limit myomectomy's complications it is necessary to perform the surgery with the correct surgical technique and in the least invasive way possible, limiting intraoperative bleeding, obtaining optimal hemostasis, proceeding with a delicate manipulation of the tissues, choosing well-tolerated suture materials and limiting the use of gauze and cloths (in the case of laparotomy surgery).

DISADVANTAGES AND INTRA/POST-OPERATIVE RISKS OF CONSERVATIVE SURGERY

- Hemorrhage (often in case of multiple and/or large myomas). The risk of bleeding increases related to the degree of complexity of the operation and the number of myomas to be removed
- post-operative entero-visceral and utero-bladder adhesions, substantially due to the trauma caused to the tissues (from ischemic damage, foreign body reaction and incorrect hemostasis); they can negatively affect the fertility and cause abdominal-pelvic pain in the long term
- persistence or recurrence of myomas with the need for new surgical treatment (reported with a frequency of 10 - 20%).

LAPAROSCOPIC MYOMECTOMY

Laparoscopic myomectomy is the ideal minimally invasive surgery for women with intramural-subserosal fibroids (FIGO class 3 - 7) who want offspring. The incision of the uterine surface on the side of the myoma implant is performed thanks to instruments that exploit bipolar energy.

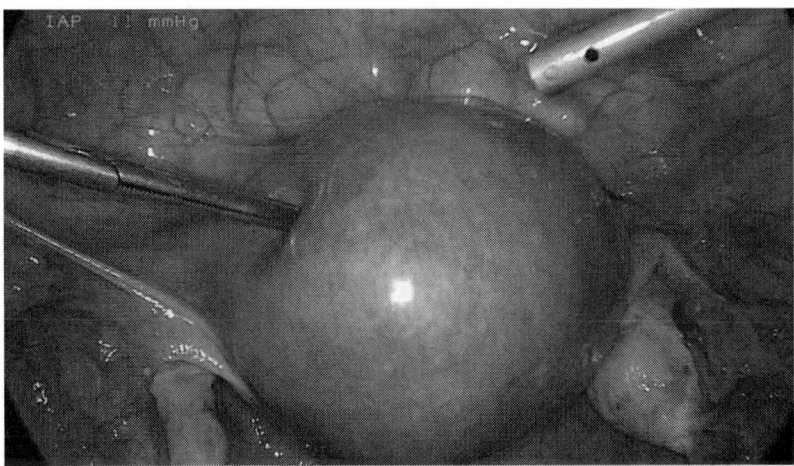

Figure 1. Laparoscopic myomectomy for anterior intramural myoma (Courtesy of Dott. Zaccoletti and Dott. Fiaccavento, EGT, Peschiera del Garda).

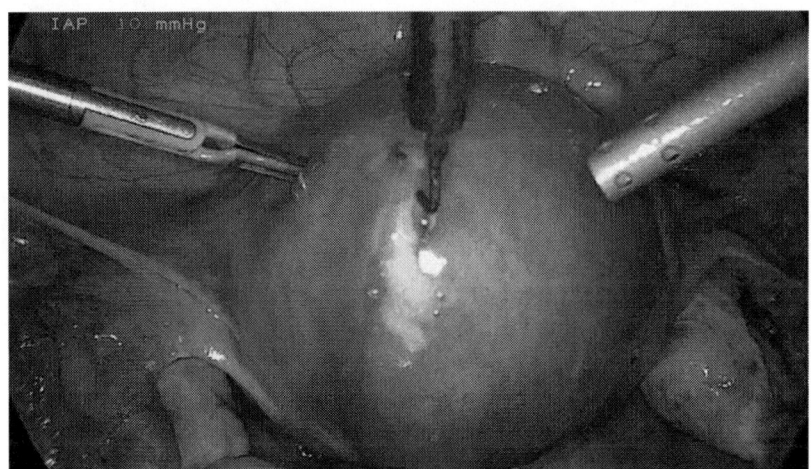

Figure 2. The incision of the uterine surface is performed with a hook (Courtesy of Dott. Zaccoletti and Dott. Fiaccavento, EGT, Peschiera del Garda).

The direction of the incision can be transverse or longitudinal: of these, the transverse incision of the body of the uterus causes less damage considering the orientation of the uterine vessels (arcuate and radial arteries).

A sufficiently large incision must be made to allow adequate removal of the nodes without increasing the risk of bleeding. Active bleeding from the incision area on the uterus is stopped thanks to the bipolar current. To reduce bleeding in any case it is necessary to remove the fibroid capsule as close as possible to the node.

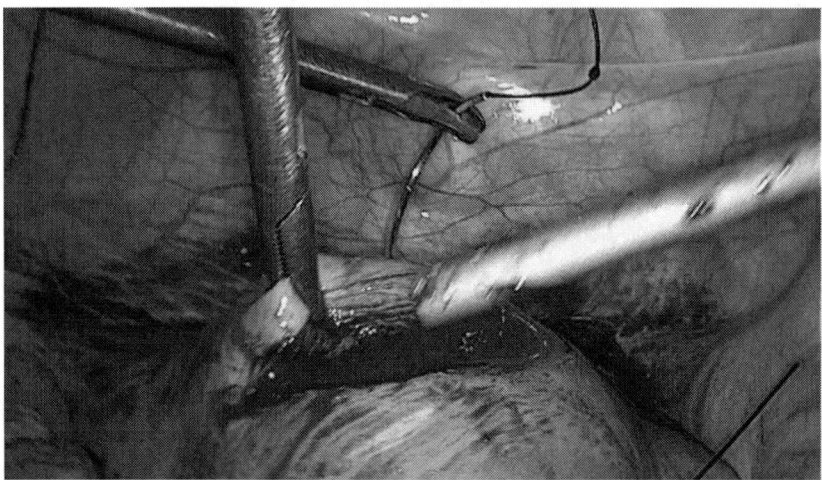

Figure 3. Immediately after myomectomy, the uterine breach should be repaired (Courtesy of Dott. Zaccoletti and Dott. Fiaccavento, EGT, Peschiera del Garda).

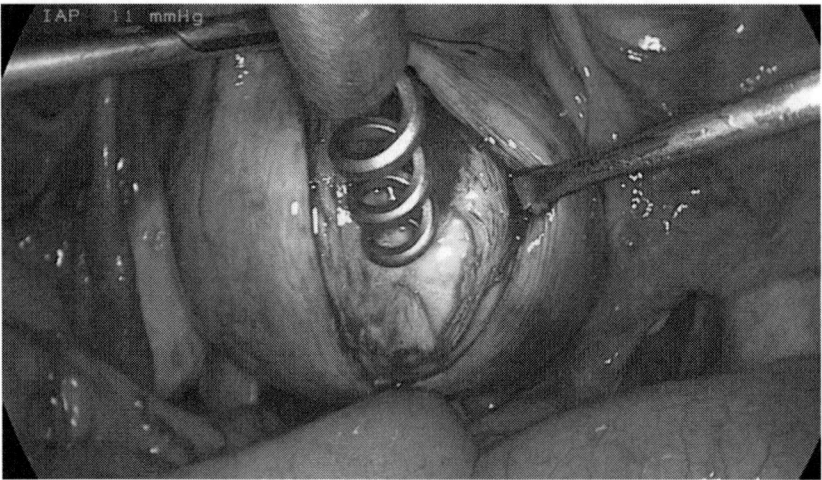

Figure 4. Laparoscopic myomectomy for posterior intramural myoma. After a sufficiently large incision, a traction on the myoma node is made with the tirebouchon (it is possible to stop or reduce bleeding by stretching the muscle fibers of the uterus) (Courtesy of Dott. Zaccoletti and Dott. Fiaccavento, EGT, Peschiera del Garda).

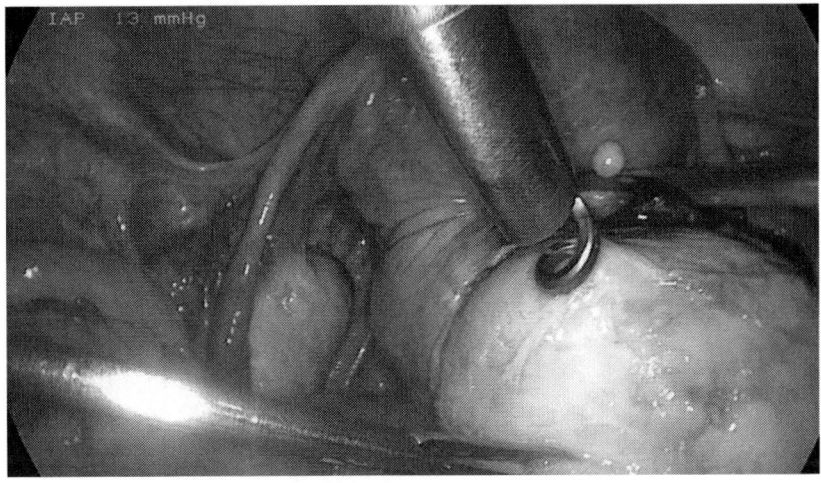

Figure 5. Removal of the posterior myoma (Courtesy of Dott. Zaccoletti and Dott. Fiaccavento, EGT, Peschiera del Garda).

Using a tirebouchon and traction on the myoma node, it is possible to stop bleeding by stretching the muscle fibers of the uterus.

In the case of large myomas, the use of the tirebouchon may not become easy. In addition, care must be taken in the case the instrument is applied too deeply or in the case that the myoma is necrotic: in the latter case, the utmost caution must be used. During the removal of large fibroids it is important to avoid damaging the endometrium: if this is accidentally damaged, it is possible to perform a continuous suture with 3/0 absorbable thread. To avoid the formation of hematomas between the endometrial and myometrial layers, the literature describes the possibility of suturing the endometrium with the first myometrial layer. Immediately after myomectomy, the uterine breach should be repaired with a 1/0 Vycril resorbable hemostatic suture. In the case of major bleeding (such as after the removal of large myoma nodes), the bleeding can be controlled by means of a Z-suture of the myoma bed.

The suture must be accurate so as to avoid the formation of a hematoma: to ensure that no dead space is created, it is necessary to check the myoma bed and suture the uterus musculature in two or four layers using Z-sutures (stitches detached or continuously) [4].

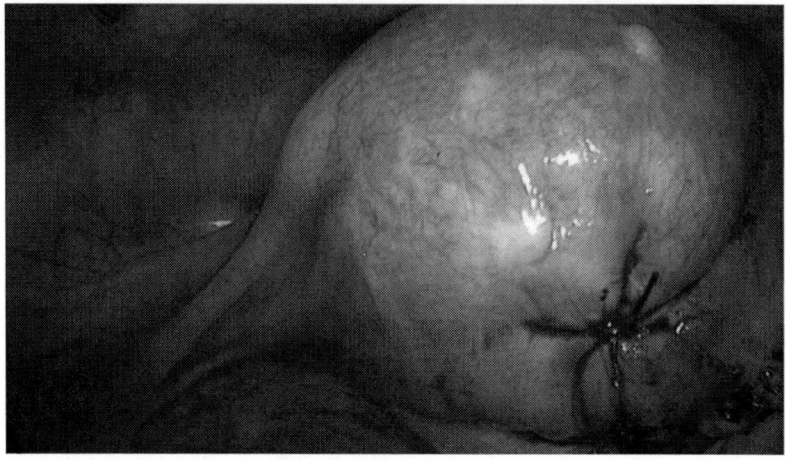

Figure 6. Hemostatic suture of the uterine breach (Courtesy of Dott. Zaccoletti and Dott. Fiaccavento, EGT, Peschiera del Garda).

TECHNICAL NOTES

- myoma enucleation should always be preceded by the intralesional injection of an ischemic solution (eg adrenaline or vasopressin) in order to reduce the vascularization of the myoma before the incision
- the usefulness of ligation of the uterine arteries is described to reduce the risk of intraoperative bleeding
- incision can be performed with monopolar current hook or CO_2 laser.
  The smallest myomas can always be treated with the monopolar current, which determines the vaporization of the water, the denaturation of proteins and the colliquation of the myomatous tissue
- the removal of subserosal and/or intramural fibroids while keeping the pseudocapsule intact allows the preservation of endometrial and myometrial integrity as well as the reduction of possible complications [5]

Surgical Treatment for Uterine Fibroids

- the removal of the operating pieces by morcellization (endobag) or by posterior colpotomy or minilaparotomy allows the risk reduction of dispersion of myomatous fragments in the cavity
- it is advisable a thorough peritoneal washing and complete removal of visible tissue fragments to avoid the appearance of adenomyotic masses or parasitic fibroids in the post-operative period.

BENEFIT LPS VS LPT

- post-operative pain reduction
- recovery times reduction
- length of post-operative hospital stay reduction (social and economic advantage)
- more favorable fertility rates and pregnancy outcomes after LPS vs LPT surgery, obviously if there are no other causes of infertility
- less time to conceive after LPS myomectomy [5]

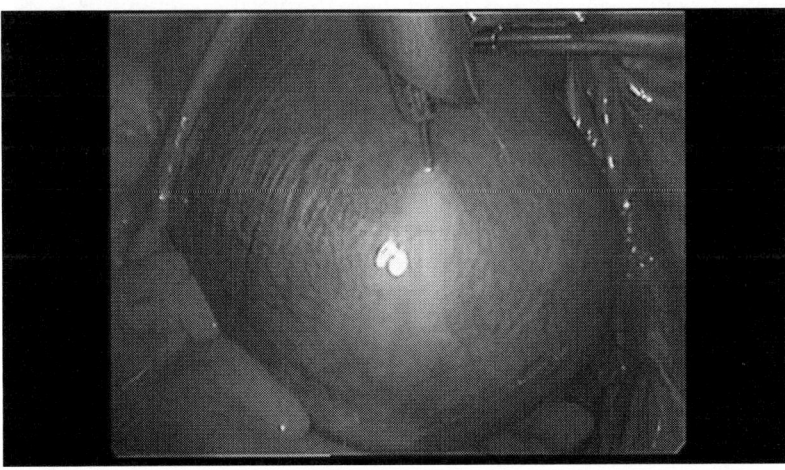

Figure 7. Intramiometrial injection of an ischemic solution before the myoma incision.

CONTRAINDICATIONS TO LAPAROSCOPIC MYOMECTOMY

- presence of multiple myomas (equal to or greater than 4, positioned in different locations) or intramural greater than 10 - 12cm (caution with fibroids greater than 5cm in diameter or FIGO 3 intramural fibroids)
- anesthetic contraindications to LPS [6]

"SINGLE PORT MINIMALLY INVASIVE SURGERY" OR "LAPARO-ENDOSCOPIC SINGLE SITE" (LESS)

The concept of LESS was introduced in gynecology in 1969, when Wheeless described single-access laparoscopy for female sterilization. In the following years, the possibility of performing more complex surgical procedures was outlined thanks to the improvement of port systems, instrumentation and video systems.

In the perspective of reducing the morbidity of laparoscopy, reducing hospitalization and improving the aesthetic result, LESS has developed in the context of E-NOTES (Embrionic Natural Orifice Transumbilical Endoscopic Surgery) surgery.

TECHNICAL NOTES

Patients must be carefully selected: patients with small myomas are ideal, therefore having to proceed with the least possible number of sutures on the uterus. The use of the uterine manipulator is of great help, being able to expose the region to be operated on to the first operator: in fact, it acts as additional forceps.

Good results have been reported in the literature on the use of LESS for myomectomy, even if the published studies are limited and with a small sample. The surgical technique was described by Einarsson in 2010: three 5mm trocars were placed at the level of the umbilical suture, with separate fascia incisions and myomectomy of a 4cm postero-fundic IM myoma was performed, with subsequent metroplasty double layer. The removed myoma had a maximum diameter of 9.6cm. The surgical technique does not differ from the traditional one.

DISADVANTAGES

The main disadvantages related to the LESS technique include the need for dedicated instrumentation, with laparoscopes and flexible or angled instruments; the coexistence of several instruments in the same site (loss of triangulation); more difficult ergonomics; need for high surgical skill in advanced laparoscopic surgery.

CONTRAINDICATIONS AND COMPLICATIONS

Contraindications and complications are comparable to those described for conventional laparoscopy [7].

HYSTEROSCOPIC MYOMECTOMY

Resectoscopic myomectomy is now recognized as an effective, safe and minimally invasive surgical procedure of choice for the removal of submucosal myomas (FIGO 0, 1 and 2) [6]. Small fibroids with a diameter of less than 2cm are currently removed routinely on an outpatient basis according to the techniques described by Bettocchi [5].

Technical Notes

1) Cutting of the base of the pedunculated fibroid with diathermic loop, possible extraction of the fibroid with ring forceps.
2) Slicing technique with one-step procedure: most used technique for the complete removal of a submucosal fibroid. It is performed by repeated and progressive passage of the mono or bipolar loop in order to remove the entire fibroid by producing slices. The operation is considered complete when the fasciculated fibers of the myometrium are viewed.

In the case of large myomas (greater than 3cm in diameter) there is an increased risk of intraoperative complications.

Two-step procedure: used for FIGO class 1 - 3 fibroids After resection or ablation of the protruding portion of the fibroid (first hysteroscopic step), the remaining intramural portion tends to rapidly migrate into the uterine cavity, with a parallel increase in the thickness of the myometrial wall so as to allow a complete and safe excision of the fibroid (second hysteroscopic step) [12].

Advantages

- effective in the control of menometrorrhages associated with the presence of fibroids
- possible increase in the chances of post-procedure conception (post-resectoscopy pregnancy rates from 16.7% to 76.9%, with an average of 45%). In fact, resectoscopic myomectomy in asymptomatic infertile women with submucosal myomas seems the most reasonable option possible. Surgical technique to be considered in case of infertility/subfertility in the presence of

submucosal fibroids greater than 2cm or intramural imprinting the uterine cavity.

Although the technique is widely described and used, there is still little scientific evidence to support its use in women with unexplained infertility [11].

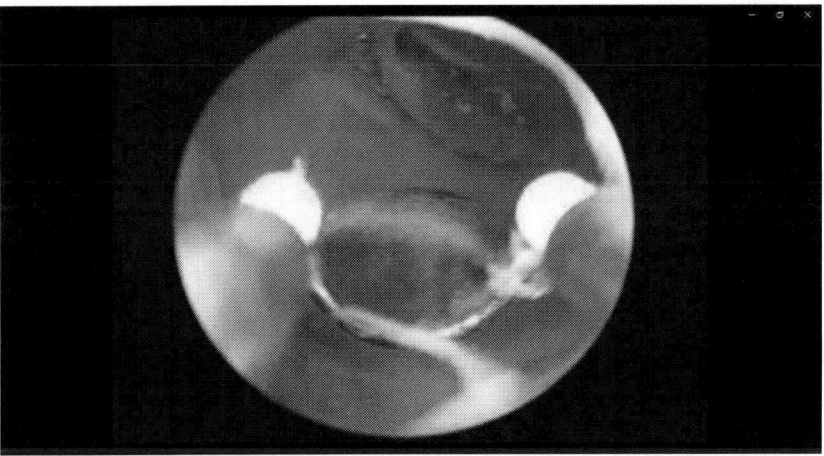

Figure 8. Histeroscopic myomectomy. Slicing technique with one-step procedure.

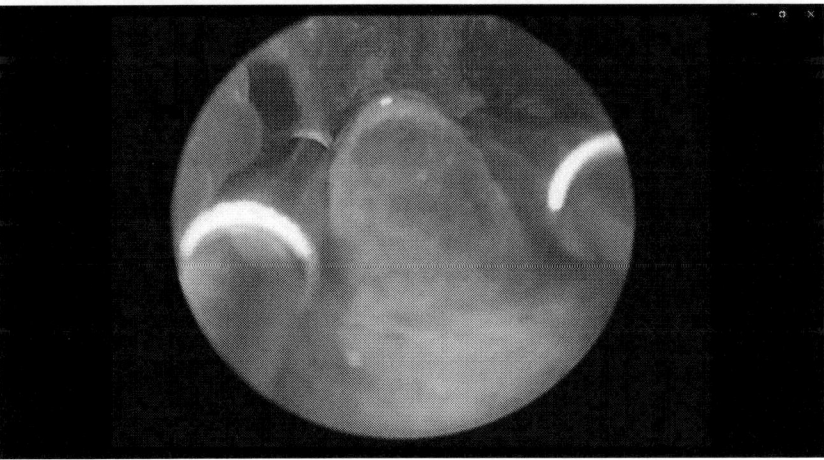

Figure 9. Histeroscopic myomectomy. Slicing technique with one-step procedure.

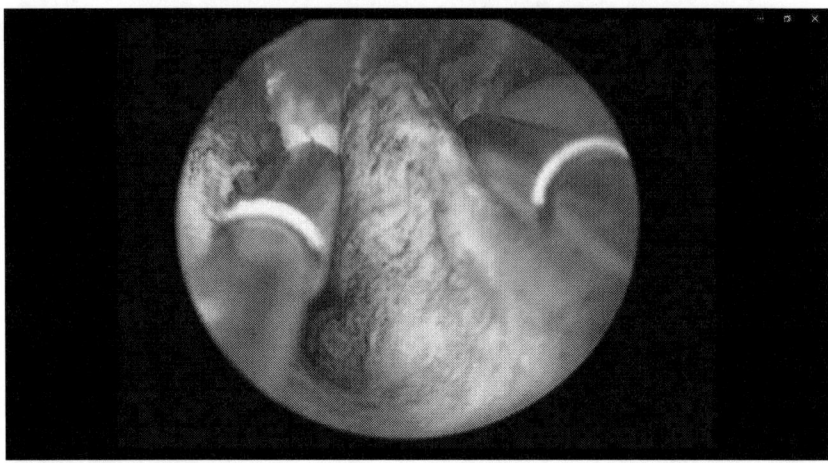

Figure 10. Histeroscopic myomectomy. Slicing technique with one-step procedure.

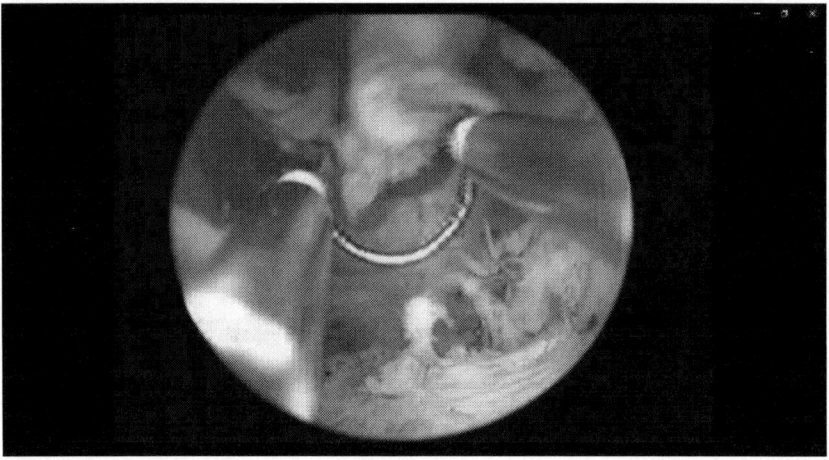

Figure 11. Histeroscopic myomectomy. Slicing technique with one-step procedure.

COMPLICATIONS

Possible intraoperative complications are hemorrhage, uterine perforation, cervical laceration and intravasation. Long-term sequelae include uterine synechiae [5].

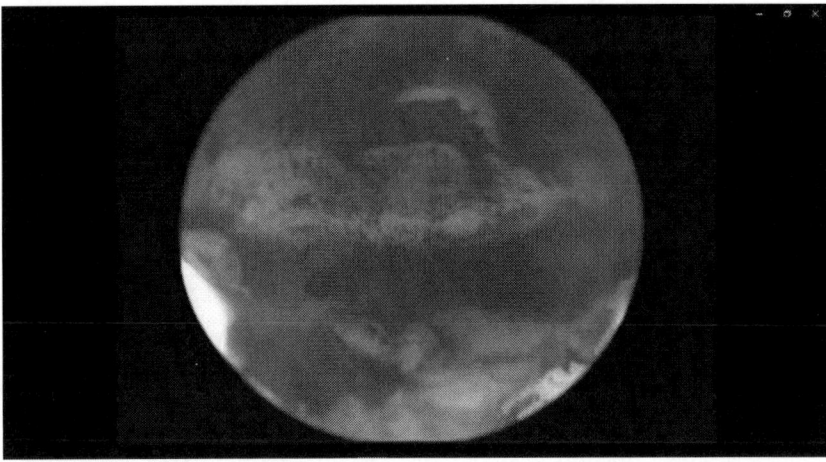

Figure 12. Histeroscopic myomectomy. Slicing technique with one-step procedure, end of the intervention.

LAPAROTOMIC MYOMECTOMY

Laparotomic myomectomy is often the only solution in women with large and/or multiple myomas, wishing to preserve fertility. The number of laparotomic myomectomies is for this reason on the rise, representing 12 - 13% of all possible procedures for the removal of uterine myomas.

PATIENT SELECTION

Laparotomic myomectomy is performed primarily in women with intramural or subserosal leiomyomas. Although the procedure of choice for intracavitary myomas (submucosal and some intramural myomas that protrude into the endometrial cavity, below 5cm) is hysteroscopic, they can be removed during laparotomic myomectomy. Suitable candidates for laparotomic myomectomy are women with the following characteristics:

- symptomatic uterine fibroids;
- contraindications to hysteroscopic or laparoscopic myomectomy;
- the need for a laparotomy for the treatment of intra-abdominal pathologies other than leiomyomas.

The most common indications for laparotomic myomectomy are:

- abnormal uterine bleeding;
- symptoms related to mass: Pelvic/abdominal pain or pressure, pressure on the urinary or gastrointestinal tract resulting in urinary symptoms (e.g., urinary frequency, urinary incontinence, hydronephrosis) or intestinal (e.g., constipation).

Myomectomy may occasionally be required for necrotic leiomyomas following uterine artery embolization. In such cases, myomectomy can be done abdominally or hysteroscopically, depending on the site of the myoma [8].

TECHNICAL NOTES

Laparotomic myomectomy is performed through a transverse incision (eg. Pfannenstiel) whenever possible.

The main elements of the procedure are:

- reduce blood loss;
- perform uterine incisions;
- remove myomas;
- close the uterine breaches.

Measures to Reduce Blood Loss

Blood loss during myomectomy can be prevented or reduced by mechanical or pharmacological methods.

Uterine Incision

The uterus is palpated to locate leiomyomas. Careful planning and localization of uterine incisions can avoid involuntary incision in the cornua or uterine vessels. Uterine incisions can be vertical or transverse. The choice of making vertical incisions prevents the transection of the arcuate arteries of the uterus, which run transversely. However, avoiding these vessels is not always possible as myomas distort normal vascular architecture [14]. Anterior uterine incisions are associated with fewer adnexal adhesions than posterior incisions [15]. However, if fibroids are found in the posterior uterine wall, it is preferable to make a posterior incision rather than passing through the uterine cavity through an anterior incision. Many surgeons make a uterine incision at a point through which all or most of the myomas can be removed. The rational for this is that limiting the number of incisions reduces the likelihood of adhesions to the uterine serosa [16]. The use of a single incision, however, requires the creation of tunnels within the myometrium to extract distant myomas. These myometrial defects can be difficult to close, interfering with hemostasis. Alternatively, an incision can be made directly on each myoma (or group of neighboring myomas).

This approach allows both easy removal of myomas and prompt closure of myometrial defects to ensure haemostasis [17].

Myomas Removal

The uterine incision is extended downward through the myometrium and the entire fibroid pseudocapsule. The plan with reduced vascularity can be achieved by extending this incision beyond the capsule, after visualizing the myoma. The myoma will then be clearly visible, the myomas are completely surrounded by vessels and there is no "vascular stalk" at the base of the myoma, as demonstrated by microscopic examination [18].

There are many techniques to enucleate myomas. Many surgeons pull on the myometrial edges with Allis to expose the myoma. Myomas are then eradicated by grasping them with hooked forceps. The plane between the myometrium and the myoma can be separated manually with the help of gauze or with scissors.

Close the Uterine Breaches

Uterine defects are closed with layered sutures. If the myometrial defect is deep (> 2cm), two layers may be required to bring the tissue together and achieve hemostasis. A polyglactin 910 (Vicryl) size 0 suture can be performed for the myometrium. The serosa is closed with a continuous suture: 2 - 0 size polydioxanone (PDS) can be used, but any absorbable suture can be used.

OPERATIONAL CHALLENGES

Large Uterus

Myomectomy can be performed safely for women with a large uterus (≥16 weeks gestation), but surgical skills and experience are required. For example, a retrospective study of 91 women with uterine fibroids like 16 weeks gestation or more who underwent laparotomic myomectomy reported a mean operating duration of 236 minutes (range 120 to 390 minutes) and mean blood loss of 794ml (range 50 to 3000mL) [17]. Intraoperative hemoglobin control was used in women with blood loss > 300mL (70 women, 77 percent) and only 7 women (8 percent) received a blood transfusion.

Submucosal Myomas

Hysteroscopic myomectomy is the procedure of choice for women with primarily intracavitary leiomyomas. For those women with myomas in different sites, including submucosal, laparotomic myomectomy is preferred. Removal of submucosal myomas during laparotomic myomectomy requires deep myometrial dissection. Often, the uterine cavity is opened. In clinical practice, the myometrium is reconstructed at the interface with the cavity, taking care to avoid the suture from entering the cavity, as this could cause a foreign body reaction and adhesions.

Infralegamentary Myomas

Uterine leiomyomas originate from the myometrium, but as they grow, they can extend or displace adjacent structures. Broad ligament myomas are common. These lesions are often proximal to vital structures such as the ureter or major pelvic vessels.

The first step in removing a broad ligament formation is a careful inspection of the peritoneum overlying the fibroid to identify a free area where the peritoneum can be incised. The fibroid can be removed with traction and blunt dissection away from vital structures. Closure of the breach must also be carefully planned after identification of the ureter and uterine vessels to avoid injury or ligature of the ureter or vascular injury. If necessary, ligation of the uterine vessels can be performed to prevent bleeding.

COMPLICATIONS

Hemorrhage

During laparotomic myomectomy the mean volume of blood loss varies between studies from approximately 200 to 800mL [17, 22, 23]. In a series of 100 or more laparotomic myomectomies, the frequency of RBC transfusions varied widely from 2 to 28% [22-24]. Increased size and number of myomas, as well as entry into the uterine cavity, are associated with increased blood loss [25]. Severe bleeding can be addressed with several techniques, including intraoperative blood retrieval, uterine artery ligation or conversion to hysterectomy. About 1 - 4% of open myomectomies are converted to hysterectomy [26, 27].

Fever and Infections

Fever occurs within 48 hours after surgery in approximately 12 - 67% of women after myomectomy [24, 27, 28]. However, a retrospective study showed that, compared to those who underwent hysterectomy, women who underwent myomectomy had similar rates of fever (39% within 24 hours), but fewer localized infectious focuses (e.g., urinary tract infections or pneumonia) [28]. Therefore, evaluation of post myomectomy fever in the absence of specific symptoms may not be convenient. Mechanisms proposed to explain post-myomectomy fever include factors related to the site of myoma excision, hematoma, or release of pyrogenic inflammatory mediators [13]. In some studies, the sites of infection in post laparotomic myomectomy have been evaluated: wound infection affects 2 to 5% of women [24, 27]; in a study of 250 patients it was found that most infections are localized in the urinary tract (46%) or respiratory tract (38%) [28].

Post-Surgical Adhesions

Post myomectomy adhesions have been well documented. In a study (n = 45) in which a "second look" laparoscopy was performed following laparotomic or laparoscopic abdominal myomectomy, adhesions were found in 36% of women [29]. Factors associated with adhesion syndrome were excision of a posterior myoma and the use of sutures. Localized adhesions, which can affect tubal fertility, have also been associated with concomitant non-gynecological surgery (e.g., ovarian cystectomy) and previous adhesion syndrome.

Others

Visceral injury is rare during the laparotomic myomectomy procedure. For example, in a study of 197 women who underwent laparotomic myomectomy, one cystotomy and two small bowel obstructions were documented [22].

POST-OPERATIVE MANAGEMENT

Routine postoperative care includes monitoring patient's hemodynamic and fluid status, controlling pain, and restoring normal diet and activity.

Inpatient postoperative care after myomectomy includes:

- pain control: continuous infusion of bupivacaine can be used via catheters placed above and below the fascia at the time of wound closure. The pump infusion lasts about until the fourth day, when the catheters are removed. Management of postoperative pain initially occurs with parenteral administration of analgesics. Another option is anesthesia modulated by the patient through a manual control of analgesic infusers. The route of administration of analgesics change as soon as the patient can tolerate oral intake, usually on the first postoperative day;
- removal of the bladder catheter during the first 24 hours after surgery;
- early feeding with a light diet;
- early walking and other measures to prevent pulmonary-vascular complications.

FOLLOW – UP

The woman is encouraged to resume her normal daily activities as quickly as possible. The decision on the timing of the resumption of vaginal intercourse is left to the patient independently, there are no medical restrictions on sexual activity [30].

Patients can return to work as soon as they have regained sufficient strenght and mobility.

Usually the follow-up visit takes place within one month of the intervention. The visit includes an assessment of potential complications and a thorough examination of the abdomen and wound. The results of the surgical procedure and the pathology with the patient are examined.

OUTCOME

Symptoms

In literature it is reported that myomectomy relieves symptoms in 80% of women [31, 32].

Unfortunately, few studies consider post laparotomic myomectomy symptom assessment, patient satisfaction, or quality of life after surgery [24, 33, 34].

Myomas Persistence

Many women who undergo myomectomy will experience uterine leiomyomas in subsequent evaluations. However, most of these women will not need additional treatment for symptoms related to fibroids. Surveillance of post-myomectomy myomas is unnecessary as imaging can detect many clinically insignificant myomas. Myomas detected post myomectomy, often referred to as recurrent, are more accurately defined as persistent or newly developed. Myomas are defined as *persistent* when they are not removed or incompletely removed at the time of surgery.

Five to ten years after myomectomy, 27 to 62% of women will present myomas on ultrasound examination [35-37]. Considering the prevalence of leiomyomas (77% in a post-hysterectomy study [38]), it is not surprising that new myomas continue to develop after surgical excision.

Development of new myomas in subsequent years is more likely in women who have multiple myomas than single myoma at the time of surgery (74 versus 11% in a study) [39]. Preoperative use of GnRH agonists is associated with an increased risk of developing postoperative myomas.

Subsequent Myomectomy

Many women with myomas are asymptomatic, so the most important outcome is the need or not for subsequent treatment after the first myomectomy. After a first myomectomy, 10 - 25% of women will need a second surgery [37, 40]. The largest study (n = 568) was a case-control study in which 21 percent of women undergoing myomectomy (open abdominal, laparoscopic, or hysteroscopic) underwent subsequent surgery within 1 to 10 years; the combination of the laparoscopic and hysteroscopic surgical approach limits the use of laparotomic myomectomy [41]. Another retrospective study of 47 women who had undergone laparotomic myomectomy showed that, on average with a seven-year follow-up, 34% of the operated women underwent subsequent surgery [42].

The risk factors for the need for subsequent surgery have not been well understood. In one study, uterine size of less than 12 gestational weeks was associated with an increased risk of a second surgery, while other data suggest that a large uterus or one with multiple myomas is associated with a lower risk of reoperation [39, 42].

MINI-LAPAROTOMIC MYOMECTOMY

Mini laparotomy is a transverse incision between 2.5 and 10cm [19]. Several randomized studies in which conventional laparotomy was compared to mini laparotomy, demonstrated an equivalent obstetric outcome and no significant differences in terms of operating times, intra-operative bleeding and hospitalization time [19, 20]. In another study, the mini laparotomy showed a perioperative outcome equivalent to the laparoscopic approach, except in the case of posterior or intralegamentary leiomyomas, for which the laparoscopic approach proved to be better [21].

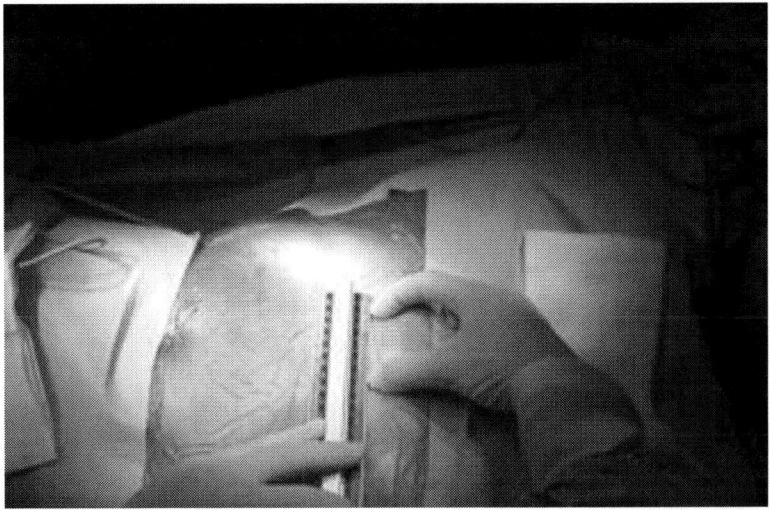

Figure 13. Mini-laparotomic myomectomy, choice of the incision (Courtesy of repertorio clinica ginecologica e ostetrica, UPO Novara).

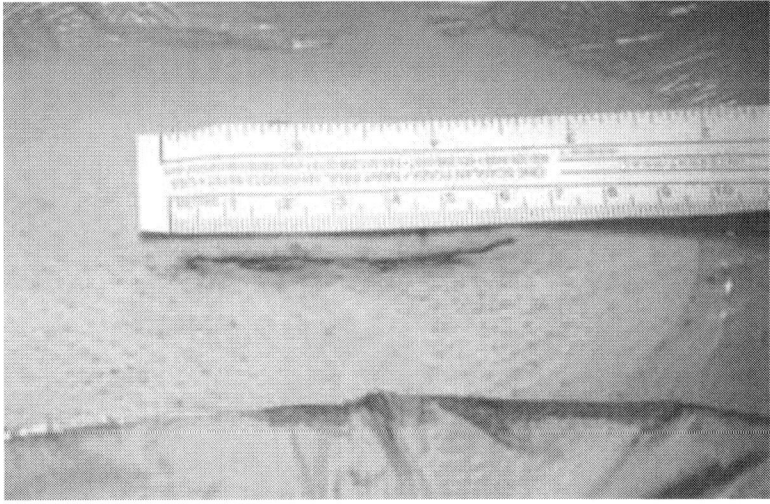

Figure 14. Mini-laparotomic myomectomy, the incision (Courtesy of repertorio clinica ginecologica e ostetrica, UPO Novara).

Choosing the operative technique it is necessary to consider the characteristics of patients and myomas: particularly the size, number and position of the myoma are the most important variables to take into consideration.

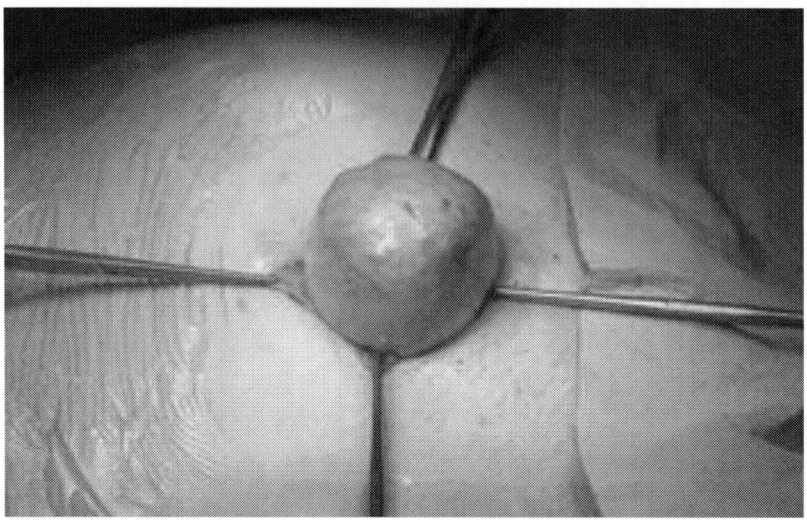

Figure 15. Mini-laparotomic myomectomy (Courtesy of repertorio clinica ginecologica e ostetrica, UPO Novara).

MYOMECTOMY IN PREGNANCY

The prevalence of the presence of myomas in pregnancy is about 2%, with a range from 0.1% to 12.5%, and it differs with ethnicity (18% in African-American women, 8% in women white and 10% in Hispanic women). In women undergoing in vitro fertilization with heterologous donation the incidence can increase up to 25%. It is likely that the incidence of fibroids during pregnancy will increase in the coming years, in association with the increase in the average age at the first pregnancy. Most women with uterine myomas do not experience any symptoms during pregnancy, while 10-30% develop complications during gestation, at delivery and in the puerperium [43, 44].

Surgeons usually hesitate to perform myomectomy in pregnancy due to increased uterine flow and perfusion. These elements increase the risk of bleeding complications and having to resort to hysterectomy, while uterine manipulation can predispose to adverse pregnancy outcomes: abortion (18 – 35%), infection, preterm birth, uterine dehiscence. Complications increase significantly with removal of intramural, submucosal, posteriorly located or multiple myoma [45-48]. Sometimes, surgical removal of the myoma is the only choice to resolve serious clinical situations [47]. The incidence of complications after conservative treatment ranges from 3 to 38% and patients who are not treated appear to have a worse outcome in pregnancy than to surgically treated patients [47].

The most common indications for myomectomy during pregnancy are: acute pelvic pain unresponsive to medical therapy > 72h, rapid growth that may underlie malignancy, compression of pelvic organs and other pathological clinical conditions of pregnancy (fetal compression syndrome, oligoamnios, IUGR, bleeding, placentation site abnormalities) [45-48]. In the past it was thought that in the first trimester the main option would be to terminate the pregnancy followed by a subsequent myomectomy; today there is evidence that myomectomy can also be performed during the second-third trimester. Although laparotomy myomectomy has been the best known method since the late 19th century, a recent systematic review pointed out that laparoscopic myomectomy should be considered the first choice for abdominal and pelvic surgery during pregnancy during any gestational age as it provides better intra-abdominal visualization, a minimally invasive approach and early mobilization after surgery (essential to prevent thromboembolism) [49]. Pneumoperitoneum induction can be performed safely by adjusting the access site according to the height of the bottom. Insufflation of CO_2 at 10 - 15mmHg can be used safely. To ensure hemostasis, bipolar electricity is the best choice to minimize myometrial damage and any possible injury to the fetus. Care should be taken during morcellation to avoid damage to the uterus or surrounding tissues.

The pregnant patient should be placed in the left lateral position during surgery to reduce the compression of the vena cava as much as possible. Fetal heart rate monitoring should be performed immediately before and after the procedure to confirm fetal well-being.

CONCEPTION AND PREGNANCY AFTER MYOMECTOMY

Time to Conception

Women undergoing myomectomy with significant involvement of the uterine wall should wait several months before attempting to conceive; recommendations for this interval range from at least three to six months [50].

Infertility

If a woman has difficulty conceiving following a myomectomy, early evaluation of the uterine cavity and fallopian tubes with a hysterosalpingogram is recommended [51].

Uterine Rupture during Pregnancy after Myomectomy

Myomectomy appears to be associated with an increased risk of uterine rupture during subsequent pregnancy, but it is difficult to establish the degree of risk and whether opening the uterine cavity increases this risk. Many experts recommend caesarean delivery as a conservative approach.

Myomectomy during Pregnancy

Myomectomy is rarely performed during pregnancy and usually for an indication of intractable fibroid pain. In addition, in rare cases, myomectomy is required at the time of cesarean delivery to allow access to the incision site on the uterus.

REFERENCES

[1] Pritts, E. A., Parker, W. H., Olive, D. L. Fibroids and infertility: An updated systematic review of the evidence. *Fertil Steril.*, 2009. doi:10.1016/j.fertnstert.2008.01.051.

[2] Klatsky, P. C., Tran, N. D., Caughey, A. B., Fujimoto, V. Y. Fibroids and reproductive outcomes: A systematic literature review from conception to delivery. *Am. J. Obstet. Gynecol.*, 2008. doi:10.1016/j.ajog.2007.12.039.

[3] Reiter, R. C., Wagner, P. L., Gambone, J. C. Routine hysterectomy for large asymptomatic uterine leiomyomata: A reappraisal. *Obstet. Gynecol.*, 1992.

[4] Sano, R., Suzuki, S., Shiota, M. Laparoscopic Myomectomy for the Removal of Large Uterine Myomas. *Surg. J.*, 2020; 06(S 01):S44 - S49. doi:10.1055/s-0039-1694989.

[5] Pérez-López, F. R., Ornat, L., Ceausu, I. et al. EMAS position statement: Management of uterine fibroids. *Maturitas*, 2014; 79(1):106 - 116. doi:10.1016/j.maturitas.2014.06.002.

[6] Donnez, J., Dolmans, M. M. Uterine fibroid management: From the present to the future. *Hum. Reprod. Update*, 2016; 22(6):665 - 686. doi:10.1093/humupd/dmw023.

[7] Leo, L., Surico, D., Surico, N. *Manuale Di Chirurgia Single-Port in Ginecologia.* EDITEAM; 2012.

[8] McLucas, B., Chespak, L., Kaminsky, D. Myoma necrosis following Gelfoam^{TM} embolization of uterine myomata. *Minim. Invasive Ther. Allied Technol.*, 2008. doi:10.1080/13645700701627522.

[9] Lethaby, A., Vollenhoven, B., Sowter, M. C. Pre-operative GnRH analogue therapy before hysterectomy or myomectomy for uterine fibroids. *Cochrane Database Syst. Rev.*, 2001. doi:10.1002/14651858.cd000547.

[10] Brown, S. R., Tiernan, J. Transverse verses midline incisions for abdominal surgery. *Cochrane Database Syst. Rev.*, 2005. doi:10.1002/14651858.cd005199.pub2.

[11] H. H. BL, J. A. MR, A. KA, C. SZ, A. E de los M., A. AD. Preoperative management of uterine leiomyomatosis using pituitary gonadotropin-releasing hormone analogues. *Ginecol. Obstet. Mex.*, 1995.

[12] ACOG practice bulletin No. 104: Antibiotic prophylaxis for gynecologic procedures. *Obstet. Gynecol.*, 2009. doi:10.1097/AOG.0b013e3181a6d011.

[13] N. M., C. DS, I. T. M. Conventional myomectomy. *Best Pract. Res. Clin. Obstet. Gynaecol.*, 2008.

[14] Discepola, F., Valenti, D. A., Reinhold, C., Tulandi, T. Analysis of arterial blood vessels surrounding the myoma: Relevance to myomectomy. *Obstet. Gynecol.*, 2007. doi:10.1097/01.AOG.0000290331.95709.26.

[15] Tulandi, T., Murray, C., Guralnick, M. Adhesion formation and reproductive outcome after myomectomy and second-look laparoscopy. *Obstet. Gynecol.*, 1993.

[16] Guarnaccia, M. M., Rein, M. S. Traditional surgical approaches to uterine fibroids: Abdominal myomectomy and hysterectomy. *Clin. Obstet. Gynecol.*, 2001. doi:10.1097/00003081-200106000-00024.

[17] West, S., Ruiz, R., Parker, W. H. Abdominal myomectomy in women with very large uterine size. *Fertil. Steril.*, 2006. doi:10.1016/j.fertnstert.2005.05.073.

[18] Walocha, J. A., Litwin, J. A., Miodoński, A. J. Vascular system of intramural leiomyomata revealed by corrosion casting and scanning electron microscopy. *Hum. Reprod.*, 2003. doi:10.1093/humrep/deg213.

[19] Fanfani, F., Fagotti, A., Bifulco, G., Ercoli, A., Malzoni, M., Scambia, G. A prospective study of laparoscopy versus minilaparotomy in the treatment of uterine myomas. *J. Minim. Invasive Gynecol.*, 2005. doi:10.1016/j.jmig.2005.07.002.

[20] Seracchioli, R., Rossi, S., Govoni, F. et al. Fertility and obstetric outcome after laparoscopic myomectomy of large myomata: A randomized comparison with abdominal myomectomy The size of the myomata may represent another important. *Hum. Reprod.*, 2000.

[21] Palomba, S., Zupi, E., Falbo, A. et al. A multicenter randomized, controlled study comparing laparoscopic versus minilaparotomic myomectomy: reproductive outcomes. *Fertil. Steril.*, 2007. doi:10.1016/j.fertnstert.2006.12.047.

[22] Sawin, S. W., Pilevsky, N. D., Berlin, J. A., Barnhart, K. T. Comparability of perioperative morbidity between abdominal myomectomy and hysterectomy for women with uterine leiomyomas. *Am. J. Obstet. Gynecol.*, 2000. doi:10.1067/mob.2000.107730.

[23] Iverson, R. E., Chelmow, D., Strohbehn, K., Waldman, L., Evantash, E. G. Relative morbidity of abdominal hysterectomy and myomectomy for management of uterine leiomyomas. *Obstet. Gynecol.*, 1996. doi:10.1016/0029-7844(96)00218-9.

[24] Lamorte, A. I., Lalwani, S., Diamond, M. P. Morbidity associated with abdominal myomectomy. *Obstet. Gynecol.*, 1993.

[25] Schüring, A. N., Garcia-Rocha, G. J., Schlösser, H. W., Greb, R. R., Kiesel, L., Schippert, C. Perioperative complications in conventional and microsurgical abdominal myomectomy. *Arch. Gynecol. Obstet.*, 2011. doi:10.1007/s00404-010-1622-y.

[26] Viswanathan, M., Hartmann, K., McKoy, N. et al. Management of uterine fibroids: An update of the evidence. *Evid. Rep. Technol. Assess*, (Full Rep). 2007.

[27] Olufowobi, O., Sharif, K., Papaionnou, S., Neelakantan, D., Mohammed, H., Afnan, M. Are the anticipated benefits of myomectomy achieved in women of reproductive age? A 5-year review of the results at a UK tertiary hospital. *J. Obstet. Gynaecol.*, (Lahore). 2004. doi:10.1080/01443610410001685600.

[28] Rybak, E. A., Polotsky, A. J., Woreta, T., Hailpern, S. M., Bristow, R. E. Explained compared with unexplained fever in postoperative myomectomy and hysterectomy patients. *Obstet. Gynecol.*, 2008. doi:10.1097/AOG.0b013e31816baea8.

[29] Dubuisson, J. B., Fauconnier, A., Chapron, C., Kreiker, G., Nörgaard, C. Second look after laparoscopic myomectomy. *Hum. Reprod.*, 1998. doi:10.1093/humrep/13.8.2102.

[30] Minig, L., Trimble, E. L., Sarsotti, C., Sebastiani, M. M., Spong, C. Y. Building the evidence base for postoperative and postpartum advice. *Obstet. Gynecol.*, 2009. doi:10.1097/ AOG.0b01 3e3181b6f50d.

[31] Buttram, V. C., Reiter, R. C. Uterine leiomyomata: Etiology, symptomatology, and management. *Fertil. Steril.*, 1981. doi:10.1016/s0015-0282(16)45789-4.

[32] Broder, M. S., Goodwin, S., Chen, G. et al. Comparison of long-term outcomes of myomectomy and uterine artery embolization. *Obstet. Gynecol.*, 2002. doi:10.1016/s0029-7844(02)02182-8.

[33] Maddalena, S., De Giorgi, O., Pesole, A., Crosignani, P. G. Determinants of reproductive outcome after abdominal myomectomy for infertility. *Fertil. Steril.*, 1999. doi:10.1016/ S0015-0282(99)00200-9.

[34] Ikpeze, O. C., Nwosu, O. B. Features of uterine fibroids treated by abdominal myomectomy at Nnewi, Nigeria. *J. Obstet. Gynaecol.*, (Lahore). 1998. doi:10.1080/01443619866381.

[35] Fedele, L., Parazzini, F., Luchini, L., Mezzopane, R., Tozzi, L., Villa, L. Recurrence of fibroids after myomectomy: A transvaginal ultrasonographic study. *Hum. Reprod.*, 1995. doi:10.1093/oxfordjournals.humrep.a136176.

[36] Candiani, G. B., Fedele, L., Parazzini, F., Villa, L. Risk of recurrence after myomectomy. *BJOG An Int. J. Obstet. Gynaecol.*, 1991. doi:10.1111/j.1471-0528.1991.tb13429.x.

[37] Acien, P., Quereda, F. Abdominal myomectomy: Results of a simple operative technique. *Fertil. Steril.*, 1996; 65(1):41 - 51. doi:10.1016/S0015-0282(16)58025-X.

[38] Cramer, S. F., Patel, A. The frequency of uterine leiomyomas. *Am. J. Clin. Pathol.*, 1990. doi:10.1093/ajcp/94.4.435.

[39] Hanafi, M. Predictors of leiomyoma recurrence after myomectomy. *Obstet. Gynecol.*, 2005. doi:10.1097/01.AOG.0000156298.74317.62.

[40] Fauconnier, A., Chapron, C., Babaki-Fard, K., Dubuisson, J. B. Recurrence of leiomyomata after myomectomy. *Hum. Reprod. Update*, 2000. doi:10.1093/humupd/6.6.595.

[41] Thompson, L. B., Reed, S. D., McCrummen, B. K., Warolin, A. K., Newton, K. M. Leiomyoma characteristics and risk of subsequent surgery after myomectomy. *Int. J. Gynecol. Obstet.*, 2006. doi:10.1016/j.ijgo.2006.07.009.

[42] Stewart, E. A., Faur, A. V., Wise, L. A., Reilly, R. J., Harlow, B. L. Predictors of subsequent surgery for uterine leiomyomata after abdominal myomectomy. *Obstet. Gynecol.*, 2002; 99(3):426 - 432. doi:10.1016/S0029-7844(01)01762-8.

[43] Deveer, M. R., Deveer, R., Engin-Ustun, Y. et al. Comparison of pregnancy outcomes in different localizations of uterine fibroids. *Clin. Exp. Obstet. Gynecol.*, 2012.

[44] Vilos, G. A., Allaire, C., Laberge, P. Y. et al. The Management of Uterine Leiomyomas. *J. Obstet. Gynaecol. Canada*, 2015. doi:10.1016/S1701-2163(15)30338-8.

[45] Saccardi, C., Visentin, S., Noventa, M., Cosmi, E., Litta, P., Gizzo, S. Uncertainties about laparoscopic myomectomy during pregnancy: A lack of evidence or an inherited misconception? A critical literature review starting from a peculiar case. *Minim. Invasive Ther. Allied Technol.*, 2015. doi:10.3109/13645706.2014.987678.

[46] Sentilhes, L., Sergent, F., Verspyck, E., Gravier, A., Roman, H., Marpeau, L. Laparoscopic myomectomy during pregnancy

resulting in septic necrosis of the myometrium. *BJOG An Int. J. Obstet. Gynaecol.*, 2003. doi:10.1111/j.1471-0528.2003.03045.x.

[47] Algara, A. C. orte., Rodríguez A. G. óngor., Vázquez A. C. orte. et al. Laparoscopic Approach for Fibroid Removal at 18 Weeks of Pregnancy. *Surg. Technol. Int.*, 2015.

[48] Bulletti, C., De Ziegler, D., Polli, V., Flamigni, C. The role of leiomyomas in infertility. *J. Am. Assoc. Gynecol. Laparosc.*, 1999; 6(4):441 - 445. doi:10.1016/S1074-3804(99)80008-5.

[49] Yoshino, O., Hayashi, T., Osuga, Y. et al. Decreased pregnancy rate is linked to abnormal uterine peristalsis caused by intramural fibroids. *Hum. Reprod.*, 2010. doi:10.1093/humrep/deq222.

[50] Tsuji, S., Takahashi, K., Imaoka, I., Sugimura, K., Miyazaki, K., Noda, Y. MRI evaluation of the uterine structure after myomectomy. *Gynecol. Obstet. Invest.*, 2006. doi:10.1159/000089144.

[51] Wallach, E. E., Vlahos, N. F. Uterine myomas: An overview of development, clinical features, and management. *Obstet. Gynecol.*, 2004. doi:10.1097/01.AOG.0000136079.62513.39.

In: Uterine Fibroids … ISBN: 978-1-53619-184-4
Editors: Marco Mitidieri et al. © 2021 Nova Science Publishers, Inc.

Chapter 6

POSTOPERATIVE CARE AFTER MYOMECTOMY SURGERY

Chiara Ferrari and Giuseppina Poppa*
Emergency Department, S. Anna Hospital,
University of Torino, Turin, Italy

ABSTRACT

Postoperative care after myomectomy surgery are given by all the involved professionals in order to support and help the patient to return to a state of health. Postoperative nursing care includes pain control, with the administration of prescribed analgesic drugs, early feeding within the first 24 hours after surgery and early mobilization to reduce pulmonary complications and length of hospital stay. In the postoperative area, together with the urinary catheter and peritoneal drainage management, nurses are responsible for monitoring vital signs, a key point in identifying clinical deterioration. Special attention is given to prevent possible complications such as haemorrhage, infection of the surgical site and venous thromboembolism, that can be avoided with the use of both

---

* Corresponding Author's E-mail: chiara.ferrari18@gmail.com.

mechanical methods, like well-fitting compression stockings or intermittent pneumatic compression, and antithrombotic drugs.

INTRODUCTION

The "Guidelines for postoperative care in gynecologic/oncology surgery. Enhanced Recovery After Surgery (ERAS®) Society recommendations – Part II" [1] examined and critically reviewed the existing evidence about postoperative care and made recommendations.

Enhanced Recovery After Surgery (ERAS) is a multimodal and multidisciplinary approach to reduce postoperative metabolic stress response by optimizing perioperative care [2]. In the above-mentioned article recommendations are given for all postoperative ERAS® items provided with evidence level and recommendation grade.

Postoperative nursing care includes pain control, with the use of analgesic drugs, early mobilization and feeding. Special attention is given to prevent possible complications such as venous thromboembolism, hemorrage and infection of the chirurgical site. Moreover, together with vital signs detection and urinary catheter management, all the involved professionals support and help the patient to return to a state of health.

POSTOPERATIVE THROMBOEMBOLISM PROPHYLAXIS

Venous thromboembolism is the most common preventable cause of death in surgical patients. Thromboprophylaxis, using mechanical methods to promote venous outflow from the legs and antithrombotic drugs, provides the most effective means of reducing morbidity and mortality in these patients. For these reasons is strongly recommended that patients should be wearing well-fitting compression stockings and have intermittent pneumatic compression. Compared to observation, pneumatic compression stocking decrease the rate of VTE (venous thromboembolism) [3] and it's also shown that graduated compression stockings reduce the rate of DVT in hospitalized patients, especially in combination with other method [4].

POSTOPERATIVE FLUID MANAGEMENT

Fluid management is an important part of postoperative care. It is possible to drink immediately after surgery and oral intake and food can be started the day of surgery, when possible. Patients can start with flavoured high energy protein drinks which are safe and can be prescribed three times a day. Moreover, these beverages can help the patients to maintain protein and calorie intake while going back to normal diet. Intravenous fluids are needed until the start of oral diet and are usually terminated within 24 h after surgery in an uncomplicated surgery. If intravenous fluids must be maintained balanced crystalloid solutions are preferred to 0.9% normal saline and a total hourly volume of no more than 1.2 mL/kg (including drugs, approximately 90mL/h for a 75kg female) should be given [5].

PERIOPERATIVE NUTRITIONAL CARE

As fluid management, perioperative nutrition is an essential aspect of surgical care. Early feeding, described as having oral intake of fluids or food within the first 24 h after surgery [1], shows multiple effects among which accelerated return of bowel activity, reduced length of stay, with no evidence of higher complication rates related to wound healing, anastomotic leaks or pulmonary complications. For these reasons a regular diet within the first 24 h after myomectomy surgery is recommended as early feeding is safe and is only associated with a higher rate of nausea, that can be controlled, but not vomiting, abdominal distension, or nasogastric tube use.

PREVENTION OF POSTOPERATIVE ILEUS

Postoperative ileus contributes to postoperative morbidity and prolonged convalescence after major surgical procedures. "It's a multifactorial phenomenon which includes activation of the stress response to surgery, with inhibitory sympathetic visceral reflexes and inflammatory mediators "[6]. Laxatives are usually used to quicken the return of bowel function, but there are no high quality data available in gynecologic surgery. The evidence level regarding this item is low concerning the use of postoperative laxatives and moderate for the use of chewing gum. These two options can be considered and although data are limited and effects appear modest, continued use of laxatives is reasonable, also for the low cost and side effect profile.

POSTOPERATIVE CONTROL OF GLUCOSE

The surgical stress reaction is responsible for the activation of the sympathetic nervous system and the endocrine responses, with a more important cortisol secretion that lead to an increase in peripheral insulin resistance [7]. Perioperative hyperglycemia is defined as blood glucose levels greater than 180 to 200 mg/dL. This is associated with poor clinical outcomes such as increased perioperative mortality, hospital length of stay, ICU length of stay and postoperative infection [8, 9]. To keep glucose levels within the optimal range insulin infusions should be used along with regular blood glucose monitoring to avoid hypoclycemia. Elements, such as early resumption of postoperative oral intake and optimal fluid balance, should be employed to stimulate the gut function, to reduce insulin resistance and the development of hyperglycemia.

POSTOPERATIVE ANALGESIA

Gynaecological abdominal surgery is followed by pain that can be severe, lead to an increase dissatisfaction, post-operative complications and increase the development of chronic pain [10]. Morphine is usually the main analgesic used to control post-operative pain, but it is related to the development of ileus, nausea, sedation, fatigue and may prolong time to mobilization [11]. Post-operatively, opioids can be administered orally to patients that can tolerate diet or an opioid IV PCA can be used until resumption of gut function. "To reduce the opioid requirement a multimodal analgesia can be used including non-steroidal anti-inflammatory drugs in combination with acetaminophen." These are effective at reducing pain and opioid consumption and improving patient satisfaction; both should be administered regularly unless contraindication exists [12]. For patient undergoing vaginal hysterectomy local anesthetic infiltration, such as paracervical nerve block or intrathecal morphine, may be effective at reducing early post-operative pain ad opioid use and patients mobilized more quickly [13]. Regarding laparoscopic gynecologic surgery, neither TAP blocks nor intraperitoneal instillation of local anesthetic are recommended on the current level of evidence. In the post-operative period both opioids or multi-modal analgesia should be given either orally or by IV PCA depending on magnitude of surgery and predicted post-operative gut function. For open surgery, a multimodal, opiate sparing analgesic strategy should be utilized. Post-operatively, multimodal analgesia should be used and systemic opioids may be given either orally or by intravenous PCA, that should be discontinued when normal gut function resumes.

PERITONEAL DRAINAGE

Peritoneal drainages are often used to avoid collection of fluid in the dissection site, to remove blood, seruos collection or infection but it does not prevent anastomotic leaks or improve the overall outcome. For these reasons peritoneal drainage is not recommended routinely after either colonic or rectal surgery [14]; little is written about gynecological surgery and no evidence has been found that drainage gives better outcomes after gynecological surgery. Therefore, peritoneal drainage is not recommended routinely in gynecologic surgery.

URINARY DRAINAGE

The placement of an indwelling urinary catheter before gynecologic surgeries is a standard method for preventing bladder injury during operation, postoperative urinary retention and monitoring urine output [15]. An indwelling urinary catheter is an invasive procedure which often results in many patients suffering urinary tract infections (UTI): 70% to 80% of catheter associated UTI are caused by indwelling catheters [16]. "The timing of indwelling urinary catheter removal is the most important risk factor for UTI as it has been established that urinary catheterization increases the risk of infection by 5% to 10% per day of use"[17, 18]. Midnight removal of the catheter appears to be associated to longer time of first voiding, but larger volume of urine was passed compared to early morning. In addition, midnight removal is associated with significantly shorter length of stay [19]. As shown in a recent single centre study following uncomplicated total abdominal hysterectomy, the removal of urethral catheters 6 h after surgery is related to fewer recatheterizations compared to the removal immediately after surgery and to lower rates of urinary tract infection than the prolonged users with removal at 24 h [20].

EARLY MOBILIZATION

Patients should be encouraged to mobilize within 24 hours of surgery. Early mobilization shows multiple benefit as reduction in pulmonary complications, decrease insulin resistance, less muscle atrophy and reduce length of hospital stay [21, 22]. Moreover, it has been shown to reduce venous thromboembolic complications in the surgical patient [23]. Every potential barrier, as foley catheters, poor pain control and IV poles should be limited and other aspects of enhanced recovery protocols must be improved [24].

REFERENCES

[1] Nelson, G A, Altman, A, Nick, L, Meyer, P T, Ramirez, C Achtari, et al. Guidelines for postoperative care in gynecologic/ oncology surgery: Enhanced Recovery After Surgery (ERAS®) Society recommendations — Part II, *Gynecol. Oncol.* (2015) https://doi.org/ 10.1016/j.ygyno.2015.12.019.

[2] Kehlet, H, D W Wilmore, Evidence-based surgical care and the evolution of fast- track surgery, *Ann. Surg.* 248 (2) (2008) 189–198.

[3] Clarke-Pearson, D L, I S Synan, R, Dodge, J T, Soper, A Berchuck, R E. Coleman, A randomized trial of low-dose heparin and intermittent pneumatic calf compres- sion for the prevention of deep venous thrombosis after gynecologic oncology surgery, *Am. J. Obstet. Gynecol.* 168 (4) (1993) 1146–1153 (discussion 1153-4).

[4] Clarke-Pearson, D L, I S Synan, R Dodge, J T Soper, A Berchuck, R E. Coleman, A randomized trial of low-dose heparin and intermittent pneumatic calf compres- sion for the prevention of deep venous thrombosis after gynecologic oncology surgery, *Am.*

J. Obstet. Gynecol. 168 (4) (1993) 1146–1153 (discussion 1153-4).

[5] National Clinical Guideline Centre (UK), *Intravenous Fluid Therapy: Intravenous Fluid Therapy in Adults in Hospital*, Royal College of Physicians (UK), London, 2013.

[6] Holte, K, Kehlet H. Prevention of postoperative ileus. *Minerva Anestesiol*. 2002;68(4):152-156.

[7] Desborough, J P. The stress response to trauma and surgery, *Br. J. Anaesth*. 85 (1) (2000) 109–117.

[8] Kiran, R P, M Turina, J Hammel, V Fazio, The clinical significance of an elevated postoperative glucose value in nondiabetic patients after colorectal surgery: evidence for the need for tight glucose control? *Ann. Surg*. 258 (4) (2013) 599–60.

[9] Ramos, M, Z Khalpey, S Lipsitz, J Steinberg, M T, Panizales, M Zinner, et al. Relationship of perioperative hyperglycemia and postoperative infections in patients who undergo general and vascular surgery, *Ann. Surg*. 248 (4) (2008) 585–591.

[10] Myles, P S, B Weitkamp, K Jones, J Melick, S Hensen, Validity and reliability of a postoperative quality of recovery score: the QoR-40, *Br. J. Anaesth*. 84 (1) (2000) 11–15.

[11] Woodhouse, L E, Mather, The effect of duration of dose delivery with patientcontrolled analgesia on the incidence of nausea and vomiting after hysterectomy, *Br. J. Clin. Pharmacol*. 45 (1) (1998) 57–62.

[12] Niruthisard, S, T Werawataganon, P Bunburaphong, M Ussawanophakiat, C Wongsakornchaikul, K Toleb, Improving the analgesic efficacy of intrathecal morphine with parecoxib after total abdominal hysterectomy, *Anesth. Analg*. 105 (3) (2007) 822–824.

[13] Hristovska, A M, B B. Kristensen, M A Rasmussen, Y H Rasmussen, L B, Elving, C V, Nielsen, et al. Effect of systematic local infiltration analgesia on postoperative pain in vaginal

hysterectomy: a randomized, placebo-controlled trial, *Acta Obstet. Gynecol. Scand.* 93 (3) (2014) 233–238.

[14] Jesus, E C, Karliczek A, Matos D, Castro A A, Atallah A N. Prophylactic anastomotic drainage for colorectal surgery. *Cochrane Database Syst. Rev.* 2004 Oct 18;4:CD002100.

[15] Rajan, P, Raghavan S S, Sharma D. Study comparing 3 hour and 24 hour post-operative removal of bladder catheter and vaginal pack following vaginal surgery: a randomised controlled trial. *BMC Womens Health* 2017;17:78.

[16] Nicolle, L E. Catheter associated urinary tract infections. *Antimicrob. Resist. Infect. Control.* 2014;3:23.

[17] Umscheid, C A, Mitchell M D, Doshi J A, et al. Estimating the proportion of healthcare-associated infections that are reasonably preventable and the related mortality and costs. *Infect. Control. Hosp. Epidemiol.* 2011;32:101–14.

[18] Givens, C D, Wenzel R P. Catheter-associated urinary tract infections in surgical patients: a controlled study on the excess morbidity and costs. *J. Urol.* 1980;124:646–8

[19] Ind, T E J, Brown R, Pyneeandee V M, Swanne M, Taylor G. Midnight removal of urinary catheters — improved outcome following gynaecological surgery. *Int. Urogynecol. J.* 1993;4: 342–345.

[20] Ahmed, M R, Sayed Ahmed W A, Atwa K A, Metwally L. Timing of urinary catheter removal after uncomplicated total abdominal hysterectomy. *Eur. J. Obstet. Gynecol. Reprod. Biol.* 2014;176: 60–63.

[21] Kehlet, H, Wilmore D W. Multimodal strategies to improve surgical outcome. *Am. J. Surg.* 2002 Jun;183(6):630–641.

[22] Van der Leeden, M, Huijsmans R, Geleijn E, ES dL-dK, Dekker J, Bonjer HJ, et al. Early enforced mobilisation following surgery for gastrointestinal cancer: feasibility and outcomes. *Physiotherapy.* 2015 May 7; pii: S0031-94061503780-30.

[23] Cassidy, M R, Rosenkranz P, McAneny D. Reducing postoperative venous thromboembolism complications with a standardized risk-stratified prophylaxis protocol and mobilization program. *J. Am. Coll. Surg.* 2014 Jun;218(6):1095–1104.

[24] Liebermann, M, Awad M, Dejong M, Rivard C, Sinacore J, Brubaker L. Ambulation of hospitalized gynecologic surgical patients: a randomized controlled trial. *Obstet. Gynecol.* 2013 Mar;121(3):533–537.

In: Uterine Fibroids …
Editors: Marco Mitidieri et al.
ISBN: 978-1-53619-184-4
© 2021 Nova Science Publishers, Inc.

Chapter 7

UTERINE ARTERY EMBOLIZATION: THE INTERVENTIONAL RADIOLOGIST POINT OF VIEW

Andrea Paladini[*], *MD, Pietro Danna*[1]*, MD,*
Massimiliano Cernigliaro[1]*, MD,*
Giuseppe Guzzardi[1]*, MD*
and Alessandro Carriero[1]*, MD, PhD*

[1]Department of Diagnosis and Treatment Services, Radiodiagnostics, Azienda Ospedaliero Universitaria Maggiore della Carità, Novara, Italy

ABSTRACT

Uterine fibroids (UFs), also known as leiomyomas, are the most common benign neoplasm affecting women, with a lifetime prevalence ranging from 70% to 80%.

---

[*] Corresponding Author's E-mail: andreapaladini1988@gmail.com.

Symptoms of varying severity are present in 50% of affected women; 25% of these requires medical or surgical treatment. The most common surgical therapeutical options for UFs are myomectomy for women who wish to have children or laparoscopic hysterectomy for women who have completed their child-birth. Uterine artery embolization (UAE), introduced in 1995, is a minimally invasive therapeutic option with strong evidence for safety and efficacy. The interventional radiologist and the gynecologist evaluate the feasibility of the UAE, taking into account symptoms, comorbidities and fibroid imaging. UAE are performed through an artery vascular access with a selectively catheterization of uterine arteries and subsequent embolization using a definitive embolic agent. The radiological outcome consist in a fibroid size reduction ranging from 50% to 60%, while bulk symptoms are reduced from 88% to 92%. The patient satisfaction rate of UAE is similar to the other surgical alternatives, while the complication rate and the length of hospital stay are inferior, for these reasons is an excellent therapeutic alternative for all patients affected by uterine and symptomatic fibromatosis.

INTRODUCTION

Uterine fibroids (UFs), also known as leiomyomas, are smooth muscle benign neoplasm of the female pelvis, affecting mostly women of reproductive age [1].

UFs are the most common neoplasm affecting women and the lifetime prevalence can be evaluated in 80% among African American women and 70% among Caucasian women.

Symptoms are present in approximately 50% of women with fibroids and could be various [2]:

- menorrhagia which can lead to anemia;
- bladder and/or bowel dysfunction;
- abdominal protrusion;
- dysmenorrhea and infertility.

Approximately 25% of women with UFs requires medical or surgical treatment [3].

Nowadays, the most common therapeutical options for UFs are surgical treatments: myomectomy for women who wish to have children or laparoscopic hysterectomy for women who have completed their child-birth [4]. In the last few years, however, uterine artery embolization (UAE) has been introduced as a minimally invasive therapeutic option for symptomatic UFs with low complications rate reported in Literature. This procedure was first reported in 1995 by Ravina et al. [5] and is now a well-established minimally invasive therapy, with strong evidence for safety and efficacy [4].

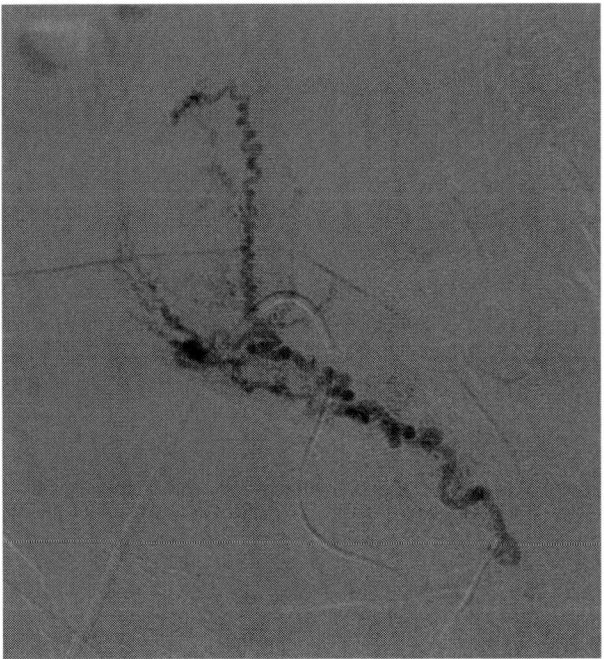

Figure 1. Right uterine artery angiogram showing tortuous spiral arteries supplying the fibroid.

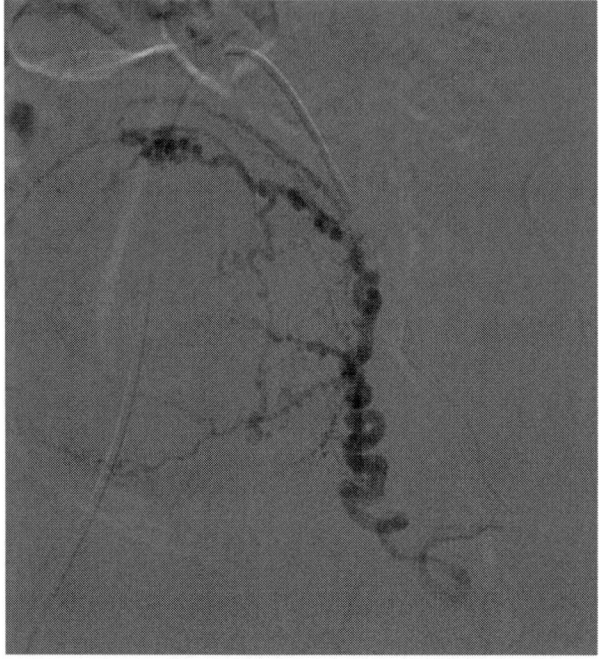

Figure 2. Left uterine artery angiogram showing tortuous spiral arteries supplying the fibroid.

PATIENT SELECTION

The feasibility assessment of the UAE must be carried out by the interventional radiologist in deep collaboration with the gynecologist, discussing the available therapeutic options (medical or surgical) together with the patient.

Indeed, it is important to consider that therapy must be individualized and should consider age, symptoms, comorbidities, number and characteristics of UFs in each Patient [6]. As a consequence, a radiological consultation before UAE is crucial so as to determinate the patient's preference regarding uterine sparing therapy, prior fibroid therapies, or desire for future pregnancy. Moreover, it is important to analyze a recent fibroid imaging of the patient, prior to proceeding with UAE.

It has been shown that a contrast-enhanced magnetic resonance imaging (MRI) is more accurate than pelvic ultrasound (US) for characterizing uterine fibroids. MRI allows not only an assessment of the pelvis and vascular structures, but also an evaluation of fibroid location, enhancement characteristics and other uterine pathologies which may mimic fibroid symptoms such as adenomyosis or malignancy [7, 8].

As far as malignancies are concerned, during the pre-procedure radiological consultation, it is extremely important to consider the differential diagnosis between leiomyosarcoma and UFs. Despite being rare (less than 1% of women with uterine fibroids), leiomyosarcoma has imaging characteristics similar to UFs. Leiomyosarcoma can occur spontaneously or could be a malignant evolution of a pre-existing uterine fibroid, mostly in postmenopausal women. Clinical symptoms are similar to fibroids, but a rapidly growing lesion (e.g., a fibroid that has doubled in size within 3 to 6 months) needs a further diagnostic investigation so as to exclude any differential diagnosis [9].

As a general rule, the majority of symptomatic patients which could be candidates for surgical treatment are also candidates for UAE [10].

The most common indications for UAE are [10]:

- heavy or prolonged menstrual bleeding (menorrhagia);
- severe menstrual cramping (dysmenorrhea);
- pelvic pressure;
- discomfort or/and excessive bloating, fullness, bothersome abdominal wall distortion;
- pelvic pain;
- pain during intercourse (dyspareunia);
- urinary urgency, frequency, nocturia, or retention.

Absolute contraindications for UAE are:

- viable pregnancy;
- active infection;
- suspected uterine, cervical, or adnexal malignancy.

While relative contraindications, requiring appropriate management, are:

- contrast agent allergy;
- renal impairment;
- coagulopathy.

Although UAE was not recommended for large fibroids (>10 cm) at the beginning, in the last few years several many Authors have demonstrated the safety and efficacy of the percutaneous procedure in patients with a uterine volume greater than 1,600 mL [2] or in large fibroids [11, 12].

Another relative contraindication, which has been now partially overcome, is the presence of pedunculated subserosal fibroids, particularly those with an attachment less than 50% of the diameter of the fibroid [13, 14].

Technical Aspects

In UAE, the operating time varies from 20 to 155 min (mean duration: 47 min), whereas the ovarian radiant exposure is about 9.5 cGy on average [6].

Even if it could be possible to discharge most patients within 24 h, hospitalization for up to 48 h is often required for the management of postoperative pain. The majority of patients return to normal activities within 1 week [3].

Traditionally the interventional radiologist performs UAE through a right common femoral artery vascular access and embolize uterine arteries (UAs) bilaterally [15]. An anesthetic assistance is required for a mild sedation.

The majority of patients with fibroids has a bilateral UAs supply. It is important to consider that in Literature, Patients with unilateral vascular supply are reported and could benefit of unilateral UAE with reduced fluoroscopy time and postprocedural pain [16].

Bilateral femoral artery access with simultaneous angiography and embolization is an alternative technique able to reduce procedural and fluoroscopy time [17].

Recently, with the aim of a fast mobilization of patients after procedure, radial vascular access (RA) has gained popularity for UAE [18].

As far as the interventional radiologist technique is concerned, an infra-renal aortogram is obtained so as to identify the uterine arteries, which are the predominant feeders in most cases. In case of large myomatous uterus, ovarian, lumbar, or other collaterals could supply the target lesion.

First of all, it is mandatory to identify any utero-ovarian anastomoses (UOA) which are the most common pelvic anastomoses. Three types of UOA are described [19]:

- Type I. The OA supplies the fibroid through anastomoses with the intramural UA;
- Type II. The OA supplies the fibroid directly;
- Type III. The OA supply appears to be from the UA.

Type III anastomosis is an absolute contraindication to UAE for the very high risk of ovarian ischemia with permanent amenorrhea, ovarian dysfunction and possible clinical failure following UAE.

Other vascular anastomoses may arise from the inferior mesenteric artery, the round ligament artery, and the internal pudendal artery.

After identifying the vessels that supply the UFs, they are selectively catheterized with a coaxial microcatheter and embolized using a definitive embolic agent (usually 300-500 or 500-700 micron poly-vinyl-alcohol-PVA-particles). Reported technical failure rate due to impossibility to catheterize arteries for anatomical variations is very low: 2%. PVA particles determine an intraluminal thrombus formation and inflammatory reaction, which persist up to 28 months after embolization [14].

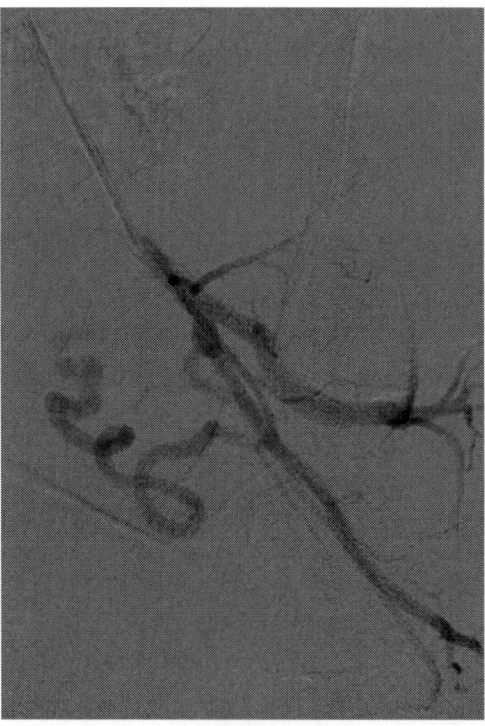

Figure 3. Postembolization check angiogram showing non-opacification of the distal left uterine artery and contrast stasis proximally.

PERIPROCEDURAL PAIN MANAGEMENT

Periprocedural and postprocedural pain management is one of the main challenges of UAE.

Following UAE, the majority of patients develop a postembolization syndrome consisting of pain, low-grade fevers, nausea, vomiting, and malaise. The onset of pain the percutaneous procedure involves 70% of the operated women intraoperatively, while more than 90% of women report pain in the 24-48 hours after UAE [20].

Nonsteroidal anti-inflammatory drugs and antiemetic medications are routinely used during postembolization pain control. Non-operating room anesthesia (N. O. R. A.) protocol is commonly used in specialized hospitals; this technique is based on the association between local anesthesia and conscious sedation obtained intravenously [21].

Superior hypogastric nerve block (SHNB) is a technique which aims to reduce the ischemic pain following UAE [20], but it is difficult and not diffuse in the clinical practice.

Some trials demonstrated that the administration of a single intravenous dose of dexamethasone before UAE was effective in reducing inflammation and pain during the first 24 hours following the procedure [22].

CLINICAL OUTCOMES

After UAE, clinical, radiological and laboratory outcomes should be evaluated. From a radiological point of view, from 50% to 60% of native volume fibroid size reduction, from 40% to 50% uterine size reduction are reported. From a clinical point of view, bulk symptoms are reduced from 88% to 92% of Patients. Abnormal uterine bleeding are solved in more than of 90% of Patients treated [6, 23]. The overall re-intervention rate during a 3-years follow-up is about 15%.

The main complications following UAE include [23]:

- permanent amenorrhea (0-3% for women younger than 45 years, 20-40% for women older than 45 years),
- prolonged vaginal discharge (2-17%),
- fibroid expulsion,
- septicemia (1-3%),
- pulmonary embolus (<1%),
- non-target embolization (<1%).

Less common complications include:

- infection,
- delayed contrast reactions,
- nerve or vessel injury at the access site,

The expulsion of uterine fibroids, which may occur from weeks to years following UAE, needs a careful management. The peak incidence for this complication is at 3 months after the procedure, with a reported incidence between 1.7 to 50%, depending on Patient selection. Pain, fever, recurrent bleeding or discharge are the main presenting symptoms [24].

Intracavitary submucosal fibroids are the most likely at risk for expulsion. The expulsion of small pieces of the fibroids is more common than expulsion of whole tumor. When necrotic components remain inside the cavity, the risk of infection increases [25].

Level of treatment required depends on the clinical status of the patient and can range from medical therapy to hysteroscopic extraction, or hysterectomy [24, 25, 26].

Fatalities following UAE are extremely rare and are normally caused by pulmonary embolism or sepsis from pyometrium [27].

Compared with the other surgical alternatives, UAE has a similar patient satisfaction rate, minor complication rate and length of hospital stay, but higher percentage of reintervention [23].

To date, there is still an important lack of knowledge about the effects of UAE on fertility and future pregnancies, in particular there are few comparative data between UAE and myomectomy [28, 29]. Healthy pregnancies following UAE have been reported but the actual fertility rate after UAE remains uncertain [30, 31, 32].

For efficacy and safety, the UAE is an excellent therapeutic alternative for all Patients affected by uterine and symptomatic fibromatosis.

REFERENCES

[1] Kempson RL, Hendrickson MR. Smooth muscle, endometrial stromal, and mixed Müllerian tumors of the uterus. *Mod. Pathol.* 2000;13(3):328-342. doi:10.1038/modpathol.3880055.

[2] Silberzweig JE, Powell DK, Matsumoto AH, Spies JB. Management of Uterine Fibroids: A Focus on Uterine-sparing Interventional Techniques. *Radiology.* 2016;280(3):675-692. doi: 10.1148/radiol.2016141693.

[3] Goodwin SC, McLucas B, Lee M, et al. Uterine artery embolization for the treatment of uterine leiomyomata midterm results. *J. Vasc. Interv. Radiol.* 1999;10(9):1159-1165. doi:10.1016/s1051-0443(99)70213-7.

[4] Spies JB. Current evidence on uterine embolization for fibroids. *Semin. Intervent. Radiol.* 2013;30(4):340-346. doi:10.1055/s-0033-1359727.

[5] Ravina JH, Herbreteau D, Ciraru-Vigneron N, et al. Arterial embolisation to treat uterine myomata. *Lancet.* 1995;346(8976): 671-672. doi:10.1016/s0140-6736(95)92282-2.

[6] Di Stasi C, Cina A, Rosella F, et al. Uterine fibroid embolization efficacy and safety: 15 years experience in an elevated turnout rate center. *Radiol. Med.* 2018;123(5):385-397. doi:10.1007/s11547-017-0843-6.

[7] Rajan DK, Margau R, Kroll RR, et al. Clinical utility of ultrasound versus magnetic resonance imaging for deciding to proceed with uterine artery embolization for presumed symptomatic fibroids. *Clin. Radiol.* 2011;66(1):57-62. doi:10.1016/j.crad.2010.08.005.

[8] Siddiqui N, Nikolaidis P, Hammond N, Miller FH. Uterine artery embolization: pre- and post-procedural evaluation using magnetic resonance imaging. *Abdom. Imaging.* 2013;38(5):1161-1177. doi: 10.1007/s00261-013-9990-y.

[9] Wu TI, Yen TC, Lai CH. Clinical presentation and diagnosis of uterine sarcoma, including imaging. *Best Pract. Res. Clin. Obstet. Gynaecol.* 2011;25(6):681-689. doi:10.1016/j.bpobgyn.2011.07. 002.

[10] Hovsepian DM, Siskin GP, Bonn J, et al. Quality improvement guidelines for uterine artery embolization for symptomatic leiomyomata. *Cardiovasc. Intervent. Radiol.* 2004;27(4):307-313. doi:10.1007/s00270-004-0087-4.

[11] Bérczi V, Valcseva É, Kozics D, et al. Safety and Effectiveness of UFE in Fibroids Larger than 10 cm. *Cardiovasc. Intervent. Radiol.* 2015;38(5):1152-1156. doi:10.1007/s00270-014-1045-4.

[12] Katsumori T, Nakajima K, Is a large fibroid a high-risk factor for uterine artery embolization? *AJR Am. J. Roentgenol.* 2003;181(5):1309-1314. doi:10.2214/ajr.181.5.1811309.

[13] Smeets AJ, Nijenhuis RJ, Boekkooi PF, et al. Safety and effectiveness of uterine artery embolization in patients with

pedunculated fibroids. *J. Vasc. Interv. Radiol.* 2009;20 (9):1172-1175. doi:10.1016/j.jvir.2009.06.002.

[14] Margau R, Simons ME, Rajan DK, et al. Outcomes after uterine artery embolization for pedunculated subserosal leiomyomas. *J. Vasc. Interv. Radiol.* 2008;19(5):657-661. doi:10.1016/j.jvir.2007.11.022.

[15] Spies JB. Current Role of Uterine Artery Embolization in the Management of Uterine Fibroids. *Clin. Obstet. Gynecol.* 2016;59(1):93-102. doi:10.1097/GRF.0000000000000162.

[16] Stall L, Lee J, McCullough M, Nsrouli-Maktabi H, Spies JB. Effectiveness of elective unilateral uterine artery embolization: a case-control study. *J. Vasc. Interv. Radiol.* 2011;22(5):716-722. doi:10.1016/j.jvir.2011.01.442.

[17] Costantino M, Lee J, McCullough M, Nsouli-Maktabi H, Spies JB. Bilateral versus unilateral femoral access for uterine artery embolization: results of a randomized comparative trial [published correction appears in *J. Vasc. Interv. Radiol.* 2010 Nov;21(11):1786. Nsrouli-Maktabi, Hala [corrected to Nsouli-Maktabi, Hala]]. *J. Vasc. Interv. Radiol.* 2010;21(6):829-835. doi:10.1016/j.jvir.2010.01.042.

[18] Resnick NJ, Kim E, Patel RS, Lookstein RA, Nowakowski FS, Fischman AM. Uterine artery embolization using a transradial approach: initial experience and technique. *J. Vasc. Interv. Radiol.* 2014;25(3):443-447. doi:10.1016/j.jvir.2013.11.010.

[19] Razavi MK, Wolanske KA, Hwang GL, Sze DY, Kee ST, Dake MD. Angiographic classification of ovarian artery-to-uterine artery anastomoses: initial observations in uterine fibroid embolization. *Radiology.* 2002;224(3):707-712. doi:10.1148/radiol.2243011513.

[20] Binkert CA, Hirzel FC, Gutzeit A, Zollikofer CL, Hess T. Superior Hypogastric Nerve Block to Reduce Pain After Uterine Artery Embolization: Advanced Technique and Comparison to

Epidural Anesthesia. *Cardiovasc. Intervent. Radiol.* 2015;38(5):1157-1161. doi:10.1007/s00270-015-1118-z.

[21] Vikrama S, Chitra R. The role of uterine artery embolization in gynecology practice. *Apollo Medicine.* 2012; 9 206-211. doi:10.1016/j.apme.2012.

[22] Kim SY, Koo BN, Shin CS, Ban M, Han K, Kim MD. The effects of single-dose dexamethasone on inflammatory response and pain after uterine artery embolisation for symptomatic fibroids or adenomyosis: a randomised controlled study. *BJOG.* 2016;123(4):580-587. doi:10.1111/1471-0528.13785.

[23] Dariushnia SR, Nikolic B, Stokes LS, Spies JB; Society of Interventional Radiology Standards of Practice Committee. Quality improvement guidelines for uterine artery embolization for symptomatic leiomyomata. *J. Vasc. Interv. Radiol.* 2014;25(11):1737-1747. doi:10.1016/j.jvir.2014.08.029.

[24] Shlansky-Goldberg RD, Coryell L, Stavropoulos SW, et al. Outcomes following fibroid expulsion after uterine artery embolization. *J. Vasc. Interv. Radiol.* 2011;22(11):1586-1593. doi:10.1016/j.jvir.2011.08.004.

[25] Radeleff B, Eiers M, Bellemann N, et al. Expulsion of dominant submucosal fibroids after uterine artery embolization. *Eur. J. Radiol.* 2010;75(1):e57-e63. doi:10.1016/j.ejrad.2009.07.013.

[26] Vashisht A, Studd JW, Carey AH, et al. Fibroid embolisation: a technique not without significant complications. *BJOG.* 2000;107(9):1166-1170. doi:10.1111/j.1471-0528.2000.tb11119.x.

[27] Vashisht A, Studd J, Carey A, Burn P. Fatal septicaemia after fibroid embolisation. *Lancet.* 1999;354(9175):307-308. doi:10.1016/S0140-6736(99)02987-6.

[28] Mara M, Maskova J, Fucikova Z, Kuzel D, Belsan T, Sosna O. Midterm clinical and first reproductive results of a randomized controlled trial comparing uterine fibroid embolization and

myomectomy. *Cardiovasc. Intervent. Radiol.* 2008;31(1):73-85. doi:10.1007/s00270-007-9195-2.

[29] Torre A, Fauconnier A, Kahn V, Limot O, Bussierres L, Pelage JP. Fertility after uterine artery embolization for symptomatic multiple fibroids with no other infertility factors. *Eur. Radiol.* 2017;27(7):2850-2859. doi:10.1007/s00330-016-4681-z.

[30] Ludwig PE, Huff TJ, Shanahan MM, Stavas JM. Pregnancy success and outcomes after uterine fibroid embolization: updated review of published literature. *Br. J. Radiol.* 2020;93(1105):20190551. doi:10.1259/bjr.20190551.

[31] McLucas B, Voorhees WD 3rd, Elliott S. Fertility after uterine artery embolization: a review. *Minim. Invasive Ther. Allied Technol.* 2016;25(1):1-7. doi:10.3109/13645706.2015.1074082.

[32] Tulandi T, Sammour A, Valenti D, Child TJ, Seti L, Tan SL. Ovarian reserve after uterine artery embolization for leiomyomata. *Fertil. Steril.* 2002;78(1):197-198. doi:10.1016/s0015-0282(02)03164-3.

In: Uterine Fibroids … ISBN: 978-1-53619-184-4
Editors: Marco Mitidieri et al. © 2021 Nova Science Publishers, Inc.

Chapter 8

UTERINE SMOOTH MUSCLE TUMOR OF UNCERTAIN MALIGNANT POTENTIAL

Margerita Goia[1],*, MD, Maria Giulia Disanto[2], MD, Domenico Ferraioli[3], PhD and Andrea Palicelli[4], MD

[1]Unit of Pathology, Città della Salute e della Scienza, Turin, Italy
[2]Department of Medical Biotechnologies, Microbiology Section, University of Siena, Siena, Italy
[3]Surgical Oncology Department, Leon Berard Cancer Center, Lyon-France
[4]Unit of Pathology, Azienda Unità Sanitaria Locale-IRCCS, Reggio Emilia, Italy

ABSTRACT

Uterine smooth muscle tumors of unknown malignant potential (STUMPs) are neoplasms with intermediate characteristics between their malignant (leyomiosarcoma) and benign counterpart (leyomioma), and represent a diagnostic challenge for both the clinician and the pathologist.

---

* Corresponding Author's E-mail: margherita.goia@gmail.com.

Clinical presentation of STUMP does not differ from that of ordinary leiomyoma, as signs and symptoms are related to mass-effect or lesion bleeding, and the imaging has a limited value in their identification. Hence preoperative distinction of STUMPs is almost impossible and generally the surgical approach is the same as for usual fibroids. The histological diagnosis of uterine smooth muscle tumors is based on three morphological criteria: atypia, necrosis and mitoses. STUMPs are referred as tumors with histopathological features that preclude an unequivocal diagnosis of leiomyosarcoma, but that do not fulfill the criteria for leiomyoma or its variants. Currently, no immunohistochemical marker nor molecular analysis is able to predict the recurrent disease. The absence of reliable clinical, pathological or molecular prognostic factors, make difficult standardization of management and follow up of patients. Current literature data recommend at least annual clinical surveillance, especially in patients that underwent conservative surgery, until ten years from diagnosis.

INTRODUCTION

Uterine smooth muscle tumors (SMTs) are classified as benign neoplasm or LEYOMIOMA, and malignant, or LEYOMIOSARCOMA (LMS) based on specific histopathological features.

Lesions showing intermediated morphological characteristics between these two categories and that cannot be classified as benign or malignant, are designated as SMOOTH MUSCLE TUMOR OF UNCERTAIN MALIGNANT POTENTIAL (STUMP).

CLINICAL FEATURES

They represent a diagnostic challenge for the pathologists and for the clinicians, because they mimic their benignant or malignant counterpart.

Mean age at diagnosis is around 50 years, as for leiomyoma and LMS and the risk factors are unknown [1]. Tumor diameter may be various, ranging from 3cm to 30cm [2]. Clinical presentation of STUMP does not differ from that of ordinary leiomyoma, as signs and symptoms are related to mass-effect or lesion bleeding [3].

Moreover imaging (ultrasound and MRI) has a limited value in characterizing STUMPs [2]. For these reasons preoperative detection of STUMPs is indeed almost impossible and generally the surgical approach is the same as for usual fibroids (hysterectomy, myomectomy, morcellation).

MORPHOLOGY

According to WHO 2020 STUMP are referred as tumors with morphological features that exceed criteria for leiomyoma or its subtypes, but yet are insufficient for a diagnosis of LMS, and behave in a malignant fashion in only a minority of cases [4].

Term STUMP was used for the first time in 1973 by Kempson to describe tumors with malignant clinical behaviour that couldn't be classified as LMS on the basis of pathological features [5].

In 1994 in Stanford Study [6], Bell et al. identifies three microscopic characteristics to classify smooth muscle lesion as benign vs malignant:

- nuclear atypia: significant (moderate to severe) nuclear pleomorphism among cells
- high mitotic rate (>10 in 10 consecutive fields at high magnification)
- presence of coagulative necrosis

Lesion showing at least two of these parameters are classified as Leiomyosarcoma (Figure 1).

Figure 1. (EE, 20X). (A) Typical Leiomyoma without atypia, necrosis neither mitoses. (B) STUMP shows focal, moderate to severe atypia and some mitoses. (C) Leiomyosarcoma with severe cytological atypia, mitoses and coagulative necrosis.

On the basis of these three features, Bell et al. recognized four histological group of smooth muscle with uncertain behaviour: atypical leiomyoma with limited experience (AL-LE: focal moderate-severe atypia, no necrosis, low mitotic count); smooth muscle tumor with low malignant potential (SMT-LMP: no atypia, low mitotic count and presence of necrosis); atypical leiomyoma with low risk of recurrence (AL-LRR: diffuse moderate-to-severe atypia, no tumor cell necrosis and low mitotic count); mitotically active leiomyoma with limited experience (MAL-LE: increased mitotic activity, no atypia, no tumor cell necrosis).

In 2020 the new WHO classification recognized STUMP-like lesion as the SMTs that is characterized by any of the following possibilities (Figure 1):

- no or mild atypia, <=10 mitoses/HPF and coagulative necrosis
- moderate to severe atypia, <= 10 mitoses/10HPF and no coagulative necrosis
- no or mild atypia, >= 20 mitoses/10HPF and no coagulative necrosis

It's necessary to pay attention because there are variants of leiomyoma that could mimic STUMP and LMS.

- Bizarre Leiomyoma (previously termed as atypical leiomyoma) that presents focal or group of atypical-bizarre cells in a background of an otherwise typical leiomyoma.
- Mitotically Active Leiomyoma with several mitoses ranging from 5 to 19 mitoses in 10 high magnification fields.
- Apoplectic Leiomyoma characterized by zones of hemorrhagic infarction.

IMMUNOHISTOCHEMISTRY

In general, SMTs are usually diffusely and strongly positive for smooth muscle immunohistochemical markers (smooth muscle actin, desmin, h-caldesmon). Immunohistochemistry is helpful to distinguish uterine SMTs from other tumors in the differential diagnosis. However, the prognostic role of immunohistochemistry in differentiating between benign and malignant SMTs is controversial. For some authors, the immunophenotype of STUMP may be closer to that of leiomyomas rather than LMS.

LMS tend to loose Estrogen Receptor (ER) and Progesterone Receptor (PR) more frequently than leiomyomas or STUMP (Figure 2), a phenomenon perhaps associated with an increasing proliferation (Ki-67/MIB-1) rate and p53-expression [3]. Retained ER/PR expression by LMS seems correlated with better prognosis and it could have a therapeutic implication, allowing adjuvant hormonal therapy [7]. Furthermore, p16 and p53 are more frequently and intensively expressed by LMS, suggesting an adverse prognostic value in STUMP (Figure 2). Ki-67 may help in distinguishing pyknotic nuclei from mitoses, with a diagnostic utility especially in tumors with nuclear atypia but lacking necrosis. Various cut-offs of Ki-67 index were proposed as useful for differentiating among LMS and other types of

SMTs; however, further validations are required and LMS may show a low Ki-67 index.

Figure 2. STUMP lesion with a disomogeneous expression of p16 (A) and patchy low expression of p53 (B); Progesteron Receptor (C) shows an intense and widespread positivity.

However, no single marker is exhaustive and sufficient to separate malignant from benign tumors. Immunomarkers cannot replace morphological evaluation and both can sometimes be unable to predict the outcome.

PROGNOSIS AND THERAPY

The term "STUMP" clearly suggests the most important characteristic of this type of neoplasms, being an unpredictable clinical behaviour. Actually, some authors would prefer to use the term "smooth muscle tumor with low risk of recurrence" [8]. In fact, most of these tumors show an indolent clinical course and prolonged overall survival rate.

In some cases, disease may recur, but usually the patient survives. Nevertheless, a small proportion of women experiences an aggressive clinical course with multiple recurrences, distant metastasis and, more rarely, disease-related death [9-11].

Estimating the true recurrence rate is challenging due to heterogenous diagnostic criteria, different follow up times and small sample size. In fact, there is a limited number of large series in literature [1, 9, 11, 12]. According to the most recent literature, recurrence rate is about 8.7 - 11% and the 5-year overall survival for relapsing cases ranges from 92% to 100% [3]. A recent literature review found 46 cases of recurrent uterine STUMPs. Relapses occur after a mean of 54 months from diagnosis (range 2 to 194 months), locally (pelvis) or at distance (mainly lung, bone, and liver). Histological features of recurrences may be consistent either with STUMP or, more rarely, LMS [3].

Although many studies investigated a variety of clinical-pathological parameters that may be predictive of recurrence, none of them resulted completely reliable for prognostic stratification.

Age of the patient at diagnosis seems to be important, since women with recurrent disease are often younger than those with an uneventful follow-up [1, 9]. Moreover, no significant correlation was found between prognosis and patient's race/ethnicity or smoking habits [1, 11].

Type of initial surgery is not a predictor factor, as several studies showed the same recurrence rate in patients who underwent myomectomy or hysterectomy [1, 9, 11, 12]. Of note, lesions removed by morcellation may recur in the peritoneal cavity, therefore such treatment should be avoided [13, 14].

Sub-serosal localization of tumor was associated with higher risk of recurrence in a single study [9].

Several pathological parameters and immunohistochemical markers were also investigated. p16, p53, Ki-67, ER and PR, as discussed above, have been proposed as potential markers for SMTs with a high-risk of recurrence. Several authors showed that strong and diffuse p16 and p53 positivity is associated with higher risk of metastasis [15, 16].

Molecular analysis tried to identify potential prognostic markers, including genomic instability (by cytogenetics), aneuploidy (by flow cytometry) and allelic imbalance (by loss of heterozygosity at microsatellites) [17].

These techniques have limited applicability in clinical practice as they require expertise and are not available in every laboratory. A promising molecular classification of SMTs using an Array-Comparative Genomic Hybridization Analysis was proposed, although histological parameters were not conclusive and showed poor interobserver agreement [17]. The authors found that a low level of chromosomal rearrangements (genomic index <10) characterized STUMPs with favorable clinical behavior, while tumors with complex genomic profiles (genomic index >10) showed unfavorable outcomes. Loss of ATRX or DAXX expression identified poor prognosis in LMS: it was proposed to identify a clinically aggressive molecular subtype of early stage LMS and STUMP.

As discussed, unclear prognostic factors make difficult standardization of management and follow up of patients.

Gold standard therapy for primary lesions is represented by hysterectomy with or without bilateral salpingo-oophorectomy. However, when dealing with young women, a risk- benefit discussion is mandatory, and myomectomy must be considered in order to preserve fertility; delayed hysterectomy should be recommended once childbearing is completed. Clinical surveillance is necessary, especially in patients that underwent conservative surgery. Frequency of periodic monitoring and whole length of follow up are not standardized and partly depends on type of surgery performed. At least annual surveillance until ten years from diagnosis appears to be appropriate; many propose a 6-months follow up-interval for the first five years. Follow up should include monitoring of chest, abdomen, and pelvis, using ultrasound, CT scan and MRI. Treatment of relapses is on individual basis: standard therapeutic approach is surgery and potential role of adjuvant therapy (chemotherapy, endocrine therapy, and local radiotherapy) is currently under investigation [3].

REFERENCES

[1] Guntupalli, S. R., R. P. (2009). Uterine smooth muscle tumor of uncertain malignant potential: A retrospective analysis. *Gynecol. Oncol.*, 113(3):324 - 326.

[2] Gadducci, A., Z. G. (2019). Uterine smooth muscle tumors of unknown malignant potential: A challenging question. *Gynecol. Oncol.*, 154(3):631 - 637.

[3] Rizzo, A., Ricci, A. D., Saponara, M. et al. Recurrent Uterine Smooth-Muscle Tumors of Uncertain Malignant Potential (STUMP): State of The Art. *Anticancer Res.*, 2020; 40(3):1229 - 1238. doi:10.21873/anticanres. 14064.

[4] *Female Genital Tumours*, WHO Classification of Tumours 2020, 5th Edition, Volume 4

[5] Kempson, R. L. Sarcomas and related neoplasms. In: Norris, H. J., Hertig, A. T., Abell, M. R. eds. *The Uterus*, 1973; International Academy of Pathology Monograph No. 14, Baltimore: Williams and Wilkins:p. 298 - 319.

[6] Bell, S. W., Kempson, R. L., Hendrickson, M. R. Problematic uterine smooth muscle neoplasms. A clinicopathologic study of 213 cases. *Am. J. Surg. Pathol.*, 1994; 18:535 - 58.

[7] Zhang, Q., Kanis, M. J., Ubago, J. et al. The selected biomarker analysis in 5 types of uterine smooth muscle tumors. *Hum. Pathol.*, 2018; 76:17 - 27. doi:10.1016/j.humpath.2017.12.005.

[8] Kurman, R. J., Ellenson, L. II., Ronncttc, B. M., editors. *Blaustein's Pathology of The Female Genital Tract,* 2011:p. 453 - 527.

[9] Şahin, H., Karatas, F., Coban, G. et al. Uterine smooth muscle tumor of uncertain malignant potential: Fertility and clinical outcomes. *J. Gynecol. Oncol.*, 2019; 30(4):e54. doi:10.3802/jgo.2019.30.e54.

[10] Maltese, G., Fontanella, C., Lepori, S. et al. Atypical Uterine Smooth Muscle Tumors: A Retrospective Evaluation of Clinical and Pathologic Features. *Oncology*, 2018; 94(1):1 - 6. doi:10.1159/000479818.

[11] Basaran, D., Usubutun, A., Salman, M. C. et al. The Clinicopathological Study of 21 Cases with Uterine Smooth Muscle Tumors of Uncertain Malignant Potential: Centralized Review Can Purify the Diagnosis. *Int. J. Gynecol. Cancer*, 2018; 28(2):233 - 240. doi:10.1097/IGC.0000000000001178.

[12] Huo, L., Wang, D., Wang, W. et al. Oncologic and Reproductive Outcomes of Uterine Smooth Muscle Tumor of Uncertain Malignant Potential: A Single Center Retrospective Study of 67 Cases. *Front. Oncol.*, 2020; 10:647. Published 2020 May 14. doi:10.3389/fonc.2020.00647.

[13] Bogani, G., Chiappa, V., Ditto, A. et al. Morcellation of apparent benign uterine myoma: Assessing risk to benefit ratio. *J. Gynecol. Oncol.*, 2016; 27(4):e37. doi:10.3802/jgo.2016.27.e37.

[14] Seidman, M. A., Oduyebo, T., Muto, M. G., Crum, C. P., Nucci, M. R., Quade, B. J. Peritoneal dissemination complicating morcellation of uterine mesenchymal neoplasms. *PLoS One*, 2012; 7(11):e50058. doi:10.1371/journal.pone.0050058.

[15] O'Neill, C. J., McBride, H. A., Connolly, L. E. and McCluggage, W. G.: Uterine leiomyosarcomas are characterized by high p16, p53 and MIB1 expression in comparison with usual leiomyomas, leiomyoma variants and smooth muscle tumours of uncertain malignant potential. *Histopathology*, 50(7): 851 - 858, 2007. PMID: 17543074. DOI: 10.1111/j.1365-2559.2007.02699.

[16] Atkins, K. A., Arronte, N., Darus, C. J., Rice, L. W. The Use of p16 in enhancing the histologic classification of uterine smooth muscle tumors. *Am. J. Surg. Pathol.*, 2008; 32(1):98 - 102. doi:10.1097/PAS.0b013e3181574d1e.

[17] Croce, S., Ducoulombier, A., Ribeiro, A. et al. Genome profiling is an efficient tool to avoid the STUMP classification of uterine smooth muscle lesions: A comprehensive array-genomic hybridization analysis of 77 tumors. *Mod. Pathol.*, 2018; 31(5): 816 - 828. doi:10.1038/modpathol.2017.185.

About the Editors

Saverio Danese MD, Date of birth: 20/02/1958. Hospital address: Sant'Anna Obstetric Gynecological hospital, SC4, Corso Spezia 60, 10126 Turin, Italy. University degree in Medicine at the University of Turin on 21/07/1982 with the discussion of the thesis "Endometrial Cancer". Specialization in Obstetrics and Gynecology University of Turin on July 1986. Specialization in Oncology, University of Turin (1991). Head of the department of oncological day hospital Sant'Anna hospital (2002-2016) Head of the Department of Obstetrics and Gynecology "A" (2008-2009). Head of the department of obstetrics and gyncecology SC4 from 2013 to present. Member of MITO (Multicenter Italian trials in Ovarian Cancer) and GIM (Breast Italian group). Author of several scientific publication in international Journals and participant in several clinical research study.

Elisa Picardo, MD, Date of birth: Torino, 16/02/1983. Hospital address: Sant'Anna Obstetric Gynecological hospital, SC4, Corso Spezia 60, 10126 Turin, Italy. University degree in Medicine at the University of Turin on 20/10/2009 with the discussion of the thesis "Risk factors for intrauterine death of the fetus: results of a study case-control perspective" and final result of 110/110 cum laude and dignity of the press. Trainee in Obstetrics and Gynecology from 2011 to 2017 in the Department of Obstetrics and Gynaecology, University of Turin. Attendance at upgrade School of acupuncture and Complementary techniques of Natural Therapies Centre for Studies and Physical CSTNF of Turin. Attendance at Consultants in Sexology course of the Piedmont Society of Clinical Sexology, SSSC of Turin. IOTA accreditation in Rome, on may 2016. Certificate of bachelor in endoscopy (ESGE) and GESEA 'Gynaecological Endoscopic Surgical Education and Assessment' Diploma on 31 st march 2017, in Belgium. Second level master in "Multidisciplinary Breastology" (2017-2018). Physician in Obstetrics and Gynecology Unit at Sant'Anna Hospital, Torino, Italy from 1 st April 2018. Member of MITO (Multicenter Italian trials in Ovarian Cancer). Author of several scientific publication in international Journals. Research grants in Gynecologic Oncology and in Obstetrics

Marco Mitidieri, MD, Date of Birth: Rivoli, 16/Feb/1983. Hospital address: Sant'Anna Obstetric Gynecological hospital, SC4, Corso Spezia 60, 10126 Turin, Italy. University degree in Medicine at the University of Torino, 14/07/2009, with the discussion of the thesis "Therapeutic strategies in the defects of the female pelvic floor not associated with urinary incontinence" and final result of 110/110 cum laude. Trainee in Obstetrics and Gynaecology from 2011 to 2016. Attendance at Upgrade School of Acupuncture and Complementary Techniques of Natural Therapies Centre for Studies and Physical CSTNF of Turin, directed by Dr. E. Quirico. Attendance at Consultants in Sexology course of the Piedmont Society of Clinical Sexology, SSSC of Turin. IOTA accreditation in Rome, on may 2016. Certificate of bachelor in endoscopy (ESGE) and GESEA 'Gynaecological Endoscopic Surgical Education and Assessment' Diploma on 31 st march 2017, in Belgium. Physician in Obstetrics and Gynecology Unit SC4 at Sant'Anna Hospital, Torino, Italy from 1 st March 2018. Second level master in "Pathways in Gynecological Oncology" 2017-2018.

Master in "Interventional ultrasound and breast diagnostics" 2016. Research grants in Gynecologic Oncology and in Urogynecology. Member of MITO (Multicenter Italian trials in Ovarian Cancer). Author of several scientific publication in International Journals

INDEX

#

17β-estradiol, vii

A

abnormal intermenstrual bleeding, viii
access, 75, 84, 101, 102, 120, 125, 128, 131
adenomyosis, 2, 4, 7, 11, 12, 13, 22, 36, 123, 132
adhesions, 27, 78, 91, 93, 95
age, viii, ix, 2, 18, 26, 28, 29, 33, 34, 42, 43, 48, 61, 71, 72, 100, 122, 136
agonist, 33, 45, 66, 69, 76
amenorrhea, 31, 63, 126, 128
analgesic, 96, 109, 110, 113, 116
anemia, 31, 32, 48, 75, 120
angiogram, 121, 122, 126
anti-inflammatory drugs, 69, 127
antiprogestins, ix
aromatase inhibitors, ix, 33, 62, 66, 72

artery, 8, 26, 30, 55, 74, 75, 90, 94, 106, 120, 121, 122, 125, 126, 129, 130, 131, 132, 133
assessment, 2, 8, 20, 21, 34, 39, 96, 97, 122, 123
asymptomatic, 24, 47, 48, 86, 98, 103

B

benefits, ix, 27, 30, 62, 63, 65, 72, 75, 105
benign, vii, 2, 8, 9, 11, 17, 18, 32, 47, 48, 73, 119, 120, 135, 136, 137, 139, 140, 144
benign tumors, vii, 17, 18, 140
bilateral, 125, 142
birth rate, 23, 24, 42
black women, vii, 2, 18
bladder, viii, 3, 48, 78, 96, 114, 117, 120
bleeding, viii, ix, x, 12, 13, 31, 32, 35, 62, 63, 65, 66, 69, 74, 75, 78, 79, 80, 81, 82, 90, 94, 98, 100, 101, 123, 127, 128, 136, 137
blood, 8, 19, 27, 29, 30, 49, 50, 53, 56, 63, 75, 76, 90, 93, 94, 104, 112, 114

blood flow, 8, 49, 53
blood pressure, 19
blood transfusion, 29, 30, 75, 76, 93
blood transfusions, 76
blood vessels, 104
bone, 22, 31, 36, 64, 74, 141
bowel, 3, 20, 95, 111, 112, 120

C

candidates, viii, 72, 89, 123
catheter, 96, 109, 110, 114, 117
cesarean section, 26, 28, 29, 48, 54
cetrorelix, ix, 62, 64, 72
childbearing, viii, ix, 22, 61, 71, 142
chronic pelvic pain, viii
classification, vii, 4, 11, 19, 26, 35, 131, 138, 142, 145
clinical presentation, vii
clinical symptoms, vii, 43
clinical trials, 29, 64
complications, viii, 24, 29, 48, 50, 52, 53, 55, 56, 73, 78, 82, 85, 86, 88, 96, 100, 105, 109, 110, 111, 113, 115, 118, 121, 128, 132
compression, 54, 77, 101, 110
conception, 22, 29, 38, 58, 86, 103
contraceptives, x, 19, 63, 66, 74
controversial, 18, 23, 28, 54, 73, 139
correlation, 12, 14, 43, 141
cost, ix, 20, 62, 65, 67, 72, 112

D

detection, 3, 21, 22, 110, 137
differential diagnosis, 21, 22, 123, 139
diffusion, 9, 10, 11
drainage, 109, 114, 117
drug safety, 33
drug treatment, 74
drugs, 33, 67, 76, 109, 110, 111

dysmenorrhea, 63, 120, 123

E

emboli, 26, 30, 31, 55, 74, 75, 90, 103, 106, 120, 121, 125, 126, 128, 129, 130, 131, 132, 133
embolization, 26, 30, 31, 55, 74, 75, 90, 103, 106, 120, 121, 125, 126, 128, 129, 130, 131, 132, 133
epigenetic mechanisms, viii, 19
estrogen, 18, 26, 65, 74
ethnicity, 18, 48, 100, 141
evidence, 22, 24, 26, 27, 28, 30, 31, 33, 34, 36, 37, 41, 42, 49, 50, 54, 56, 57, 66, 87, 101, 103, 105, 106, 107, 110, 111, 112, 113, 114, 116, 120, 121, 129
evolution, 115, 123
excision, 86, 94, 95, 97
exposure, 18, 26, 124
expulsion, 66, 128, 132
extracellular matrix (ECM), ix, 11, 33, 44

F

fertility, viii, ix, 18, 22, 23, 24, 26, 48, 62, 69, 70, 72, 74, 78, 83, 89, 95, 105, 129, 133, 142, 144
fertility rate, 83, 129
fertility sparing, viii
fertilization, 37, 43, 100
fetal demise, 50
fetal growth, 50
fetus, 51, 53, 54, 101
fibroids, vii, viii, ix, 2, 6, 7, 8, 9, 11, 17, 18, 19, 26, 30, 34, 36, 37, 38, 40, 43, 44, 47, 48, 49, 50, 52, 53, 54, 56, 57, 58, 72, 73, 75, 76, 78, 81, 82, 83, 84, 85, 86, 87, 91, 97, 100, 103, 106, 108, 119, 120, 123, 124, 125, 128, 129, 130, 131, 132, 133, 136, 137

FIGO, 4, 12, 21, 27, 32, 35, 72, 78, 84, 85, 86
fluid, 4, 95, 111, 112, 114
formation, 8, 19, 29, 55, 81, 93, 104, 126

G

gastrointestinal tract, 90
gene expression, 22
general anesthesia, 77
genetic factors, vii
genetic variants, viii
genomic instability, 141
gestation, 24, 25, 53, 92, 100
GnRH, 31, 33, 43, 61, 63, 64, 65, 66, 69, 71, 75, 76, 97, 103
gonadal hormones, vii, ix
gonadotropin-releasing hormone, ix, 31, 45, 70, 74, 75, 104
gonadotropin-releasing hormone analogs, ix
growth, ix, 2, 9, 11, 15, 19, 22, 24, 31, 33, 39, 44, 49, 50, 54, 101
growth factor, 22, 33, 44
guidelines, 40, 55, 130, 132
gynecologist, 120, 122

H

health, ix, 12, 62, 72, 109, 110
health status, 12
hematoma, 29, 55, 81, 94
hemoglobin, 28, 32, 93
hemorrhage, 9, 25, 29, 41, 48, 49, 52, 55, 88
hemostasis, 53, 54, 78, 91, 92, 101
human chorionic gonadotropin, 49
hysterectomy, ix, 10, 26, 29, 48, 53, 69, 70, 73, 74, 77, 94, 97, 100, 103, 104, 105, 106, 113, 114, 116, 117, 120, 121, 128, 137, 141, 142

I

incidence, vii, 19, 29, 30, 34, 48, 53, 100, 101, 116, 128
industrialized societies, 77
infection, 27, 77, 95, 100, 109, 110, 112, 114, 124, 128
infertility, 17, 22, 27, 28, 29, 33, 36, 72, 73, 83, 86, 87, 103, 106, 108, 120, 133
inflammatory mediators, 95, 112
injury, iv, 19, 33, 44, 94, 95, 101, 114, 128

L

laparoscopic surgery, 29, 85
laparoscopy, 26, 27, 28, 42, 73, 84, 85, 95, 104
laparotomy, 26, 28, 73, 78, 90, 98, 101
leiomyoma, vii, ix, 2, 9, 11, 14, 22, 33, 34, 38, 39, 42, 43, 44, 45, 48, 58, 63, 69, 73, 107, 136, 137, 138, 139, 144
leiomyoma incidence, vii
leiomyomata, viii, 7, 10, 34, 35, 40, 57, 58, 69, 103, 104, 106, 107, 129, 130, 132, 133
lesions, 4, 5, 8, 10, 19, 26, 93, 141, 142, 145
leuprolide acetate, ix, 61, 63, 64, 69, 72
levonorgestrel re leasing intrauterine devic, x
liver, 33, 44, 65, 141
liver transplant, 33
liver transplantation, 33
local anesthesia, 127

M

magnetic resonance, 8, 14, 20, 74, 123, 130
magnetic resonance imaging, 14, 20, 123, 130
majority, 48, 52, 123, 125, 127

malignant tumors, 9, 11
management, viii, ix, x, 15, 18, 26, 27, 32, 33, 36, 40, 42, 43, 44, 48, 54, 56, 62, 63, 69, 70, 72, 103, 104, 105, 106, 108, 109, 110, 111, 124, 128, 136, 142
mass, viii, 7, 9, 10, 19, 74, 90, 136, 137
medical, viii, ix, 12, 32, 33, 43, 44, 61, 62, 63, 64, 66, 67, 70, 71, 72, 74, 96, 101, 120, 121, 122, 128
menopause, viii, ix, 2, 18, 31, 35, 61, 69, 71
menorrhagia, 63, 70, 120, 123
mesenchymal cell, vii
meta-analysis, 25, 27, 37, 39, 40, 41, 42, 76
miscarriage, 23, 25, 28, 29, 30, 48, 50, 56, 72
morbidity, 24, 49, 56, 84, 105, 110, 112, 117
myoma therapy, viii
myomectomy, vi, viii, ix, 8, 21, 24, 26, 27, 28, 29, 30, 31, 41, 42, 43, 48, 53, 54, 55, 56, 57, 58, 59, 73, 74, 75, 76, 77, 78, 79, 80, 81, 83, 84, 85, 86, 87, 88, 89, 90, 91, 92, 93, 94, 95, 96, 97, 98, 99, 100, 101, 102, 103, 104, 105, 106, 107, 108, 109, 111, 120, 121, 129, 133, 137, 141, 142

N

nasogastric tube, 112
natural compound, 62, 72
nausea, 112, 113, 116, 127
necrosis, 3, 7, 9, 54, 103, 108, 136, 137, 138, 139
neoplasm, 119, 120, 136
non-steroidal anti-inflammatory drugs, 113

O

obstetrical complications, viii
oral contraceptives, x, 19, 63
ovarian cancer, 73
ovaries, 8, 73
ovulation, 31

P

pain, viii, 30, 48, 50, 54, 65, 66, 73, 74, 75, 78, 83, 90, 95, 96, 101, 102, 109, 110, 113, 115, 116, 123, 125, 127, 132
pain management, 127
pathogenesis, vii, 18, 33, 44
pathology, 2, 4, 7, 96
pelvic ultrasound, 73, 123
pelvis, 3, 120, 123, 141, 142
placebo, 45, 63, 64, 69, 76, 117
placenta, 25, 26, 39, 47, 48, 49, 52, 54, 56
placenta previa, 25, 39
placental abruption, 48, 50, 56
pregnancy, 2, 22, 23, 24, 25, 27, 28, 29, 30, 31, 38, 39, 41, 42, 47, 48, 49, 50, 51, 53, 54, 55, 56, 57, 58, 74, 77, 83, 86, 100, 101, 102, 107, 108, 122, 124
premature contraction, 25
pre-menopausal, ix, 62
preterm delivery, 28, 29, 50
progesterone, vii, ix, 26, 31, 32, 43, 44, 65, 139
progestin, x, 63
prognosis, 139, 141, 142
prophylaxis, 53, 77, 104, 118
prostaglandins, 25, 55, 62
pulmonary embolism, 129

Q

quality of life, viii, 30, 48, 65, 97

R

receptor, ix, 31, 32, 33, 43, 44, 49
recommendations, iv, 102, 110, 115

Index

recovery, 83, 115, 116
recurrence, viii, 30, 78, 106, 107, 138, 140, 141
reproductive age, 2, 12, 17, 18, 29, 32, 42, 56, 65, 77, 105, 120
risk, viii, ix, 2, 18, 19, 23, 25, 29, 34, 40, 44, 47, 48, 49, 50, 52, 53, 55, 56, 58, 59, 61, 71, 72, 73, 75, 76, 77, 78, 79, 82, 83, 86, 97, 98, 100, 102, 107, 114, 118, 126, 128, 130, 136, 141, 142, 144
risk factors, 18, 55, 56, 59, 73, 98, 136

S

safety, 42, 45, 65, 75, 120, 121, 124, 129, 130
selective estrogen receptor modulator, 67
selective progesterone receptor modulators (SPRMs), ix, 31, 43, 62, 65, 72
smooth muscle, vi, vii, 6, 19, 22, 34, 120, 129, 135, 136, 137, 138, 139, 140, 143, 144, 145
spontaneous abortion, 18, 23, 25
spontaneous pregnancy, 24
surgical intervention, 26, 55
surgical removal, 101
surgical technique, 30, 78, 85
suture, 29, 55, 78, 81, 82, 85, 92, 93
sympathetic nervous system, 112
symptoms, viii, ix, 30, 35, 48, 61, 62, 63, 65, 66, 67, 71, 73, 74, 90, 94, 97, 100, 120, 122, 123, 127, 128, 136, 137
syndrome, 18, 27, 95, 101, 127

T

techniques, 30, 35, 55, 85, 92, 94, 142
therapy, vii, viii, ix, 27, 31, 32, 33, 43, 61, 62, 63, 65, 69, 71, 74, 75, 76, 101, 103, 121, 122, 128, 139, 142
tranexamic acid, x, 61, 63, 71, 74

treatment, vii, viii, ix, x, 8, 12, 18, 26, 31, 32, 33, 37, 40, 43, 44, 54, 62, 64, 65, 66, 67, 70, 72, 73, 74, 76, 78, 90, 97, 98, 101, 104, 120, 121, 123, 128, 129, 141
trial, 30, 33, 45, 48, 56, 57, 70, 115, 117, 118, 131, 132
tumors, 7, 9, 11, 13, 14, 15, 34, 45, 129, 135, 136, 137, 139, 140, 142, 143, 145

U

ultrasonography, 8, 14, 20
ultrasound, 2, 3, 5, 6, 7, 8, 20, 27, 30, 34, 36, 49, 52, 56, 72, 73, 74, 75, 97, 130, 137, 142
urinary retention, 114
urinary tract, 94, 114, 117
urinary tract infection, 94, 114, 117
uterine bleeding, ix, x, 12, 13, 35, 62, 63, 69, 74, 90, 127
uterine fibroids (UFs), v, vi, vii, ix, x, 2, 26, 34, 35, 36, 38, 41, 42, 43, 44, 45, 47, 48, 49, 52, 56, 57, 61, 62, 63, 64, 65, 66, 67, 68, 70, 71, 90, 93, 103, 104, 105, 106, 107, 119, 120, 121, 122, 123, 126, 128, 129, 131
uterus, vii, 2, 3, 4, 8, 10, 11, 12, 13, 14, 20, 21, 25, 29, 35, 36, 39, 51, 52, 55, 56, 74, 75, 76, 79, 80, 81, 84, 91, 92, 98, 101, 102, 125, 129, 143

V

vascular surgery, 116
vascularization, 5, 22, 25, 32, 49, 82
vessels, 8, 54, 79, 91, 92, 93, 94, 126
visualization, 3, 21, 30, 73, 101
vitamin D, 67
vomiting, 112, 116, 127

W

white women, viii, 18, 34, 48
wound healing, 111
wound infection, 95

Y

young women, 142